Neonatal Head and Spine Ultrasonography

Andrea Poretti
Thierry A.G.M. Huisman
Editors

Neonatal Head and Spine Ultrasonography

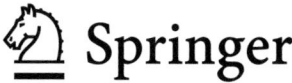 Springer

Editors
Andrea Poretti, MD
Assistant Professor of
  Radiology
Head of Pediatric
  Neuroradiology
Research Division of Pediatric
  Radiology and Pediatric
  Neuroradiology
Department of Radiology
  and Radiological Sciences
The Johns Hopkins Hospital
Baltimore, MD, USA

Thierry A.G.M. Huisman, MD,
  FICIS, EQNR
Professor of Radiology,
  Pediatrics, Neurology
  and Neurosurgery
Chairman, Department
  of Imaging and Imaging Science
Johns Hopkins Bayview
  Medical Center
Baltimore, MD, USA

Director, Division of Pediatric
  Radiology and Pediatric
  Neuroradiology
The Johns Hopkins Hospital
Baltimore, MD, USA

ISBN 978-3-319-14567-9   ISBN 978-3-319-14568-6   (eBook)
DOI 10.1007/978-3-319-14568-6

Library of Congress Control Number: 2015947271

Springer Cham Heidelberg New York Dordrecht London

Springer International Publishing AG Switzerland is part of Springer Science+Business Media (www.springer.com)

Preface

Head and spine ultrasonography is an important tool in the initial evaluation of intracranial and intraspinal abnormalities in newborns. Ultrasonography is an incredibly versatile bedside imaging tool in detecting brain and spine abnormalities in neonates, following the course of these lesions, and evaluating the maturation of the neonatal brain and spine. We believe it is a safe and cost-efficient alternative to magnetic resonance imaging and computed tomography in many cases.

This book allows readers to explore and advance their knowledge with neonatal head and spine ultrasonography and its application to a variety of common and rare neonatal neurologic disorders. Organized to correspond to daily routine bedside practice, it presents a symptom-based approach and classifies neonatal neurologic disorders at presentation. For each symptom or finding, we present exemplary clinical cases from our routine practice and illustrate how head and spine ultrasonography may help in making the correct diagnosis.

For the creation of the valuable collection of cases, we are grateful to our coauthors, Drs. Frances J. Northington, Güneş Orman, and Jacqueline Salas, who helped us with their interest and expertise in this field to select the most interesting and didactic cases and prepare succinct clinical vignettes as well as illustrative, high-quality images. To be able to complete this book, we were supported and intellectually challenged by a number of brilliant physicians who are members of the Neurosciences Intensive Care Nursery Program at the Johns Hopkins Hospital, with their professional requests and stimulating discussions at our weekly joint neonatal neurology conference. This interdisciplinary culture has its roots in Johns Hopkins' four core values: excellence and discovery, leadership and integrity, diversity and inclusion, and respect and collegiality. These are as valid today as they were at the founding of our hospital and our school of medicine in the late nineteenth century.

We are thankful to Springer International Publishing AG, who gave us the opportunity to publish our experiences with neonatal head ultrasonography. We are particularly grateful to Janet Foltin, Senior Editor, and Patrick Carr, Project Coordinator, for their support in the conceptualization, preparation, and realization of this book.

We hope that this book and case collection is as enjoyable and helpful for readers as its preparation was for us.

Baltimore, MD, USA   Andrea Poretti, MD
                                   Thierry A.G.M. Huisman,
                                       MD, FICIS, EQNR

Contents

Contributors

Thierry A.G.M. Huisman, MD, FICIS, EQNR Professor of Radiology, Pediatrics, Neurology and Neurosurgery, Chairman, Department of Imaging and Imaging Science, Johns Hopkins Bayview Medical Center, Baltimore, MD, USA

Director, Division of Pediatric Radiology and Pediatric Neuroradiology, The Johns Hopkins Hospital, Baltimore, MD, USA

Section of Pediatric Neuroradiology, Division of Pediatric Radiology, Russell H. Morgan

Frances J. Northington, MD Division of Neonatology, Department of Pediatrics, The Johns Hopkins Hospital, Baltimore, MD, USA

Güneş Orman, MD Section of Pediatric Neuroradiology, Division of Pediatric Radiology, Russell H. Morgan Department of Radiology, The Johns Hopkins Hospital, Baltimore, MD, USA

Andrea Poretti, MD Research Division of Pediatric Radiology and Pediatric Neuroradiology, Department of Radiology and Radiological Sciences, The Johns Hopkins Hospital, Baltimore, MD, USA

Jacqueline Salas, MD Division of Neonatology, Department of Pediatrics, The Johns Hopkins Hospital, Baltimore, MD, USA

Chapter 1
Introduction

Ultrasonography (US) is a safe imaging modality that does not require sedation and can be performed bedside. It can be repeated as often as necessary because of the lack of ionizing radiation. Modern "high-end" (i.e., technologically advanced, up-to-date) US units can obtain two- and three-dimensional (3-D) images of the neonatal brain in high resolution (Daneman et al. 2006; Govaert and de Vries 2010; Maalouf et al. 2001; Orman et al. 2015; van Wezel-Meijler et al. 2010). Neonatal US requires a well-trained sonographer or radiologist familiar with neonatal pathology who is able to perform an optimized, personalized study and knows how to take full advantage of new technical developments (Benson et al. 2002; Daneman et al. 2006; Di Salvo 2001; Leijser et al. 2006; Nwafor-Anene et al. 2003; Steggerda et al. 2009; van Wezel-Meijler et al. 2010; Ladino Torres and DiPietro 2014).

In the past, US has often been considered inferior to the competing cross-sectional imaging modalities of computed tomography (CT) and magnetic resonance imaging (MRI). However, many of the studies that compared US with CT and/or MRI used only limited "low-end" US studies with "high-end" CT/MRI studies or compared an acute US with a follow-up CT/MRI study done at a time when the findings were more apparent or better demarcated due to ongoing tissue injury or lesion evolution (Daneman et al. 2006; Leijser et al. 2006; Maalouf et al. 2001). It is our experience

© Springer International Publishing Switzerland 2016
A. Poretti, T.A.G.M. Huisman (eds.), *Neonatal Head and Spine Ultrasonography*, DOI 10.1007/978-3-319-14568-6_1

that a "high-end" US, utilizing modern equipment that includes gray-scale anatomical and color-coded duplex Doppler techniques, performed by a skilled sonographer, can be a very valuable and cost-efficient alternative to CT and MRI in both the acute and chronic phases of neonatal brain and spine pathology.

In this short book, we will discuss the standard, up-to-date US techniques available, how to perform the study, and what to look for on the images. We will present a variety of brain and spine findings that may be encountered including complications of prematurity, hypoxic ischemic brain injury, neonatal stroke, infections, malformations, neoplasms, and several rare neonatal pathologies. There are textbooks that provide an invaluable overview of the US findings in several neonatal neurologic diseases (Govaert and de Vries 2010). The newborns, however, do not present with a diagnosis, but with symptoms and findings, which typically guide clinicians to finally determine the diagnosis and start the therapy. Therefore, we have prioritized a symptom/finding-based approach for our book and classified the neonatal neurology diseases based on the symptoms/findings at presentation.

References

Benson JE, Bischop MR, Cohen HL. Intracranial neonatal neuro-sonography: an update. Ultrasound Q. 2002;18:89–114.

Daneman A, Epelman M, Blaser S, Jarrin JR. Imaging of the brain in full-term neonates: does sonography still play a role? Pediatr Radiol. 2006;36:636–46.

Di Salvo DN. A new view of the neonatal brain: clinical utility of supplemental neurologic US imaging windows. Radiographics. 2001;21:943–55.

Govaert P, de Vries LS. An atlas of neonatal brain sonography. London: Mac Keith Press; 2010.

Ladino Torres MF, DiPietro MA. Spine ultrasound imaging in the newborn. Semin Ultrasound CT MR. 2014;35:652–61.

Leijser LM, de Vries LS, Cowan FM. Using cerebral ultrasound effectively in the newborn infant. Early Hum Dev. 2006;82: 827–35.

Maalouf EF, Duggan PJ, Counsell SJ, Rutherford MA, Cowan F, Azzopardi D, Edwards AD. Comparison of findings on cranial ultrasound and magnetic resonance imaging in preterm infants. Pediatrics. 2001;107:719–27.

Nwafor-Anene VN, DeCristofaro JD, Baumgart S. Serial head ultrasound studies in preterm infants: how many normal studies does one infant need to exclude significant abnormalities? J Perinatol. 2003;23:104–10.

Orman G, Benson JE, Kweldam CF, Bosemani T, Tekes A, de Jong MR, et al. Neonatal head ultrasonography today: a powerful imaging tool! J Neuroimaging. 2015;25(1):31–55. doi:10.1111/jon.12108.

Steggerda SJ, Leijser LM, Walther FJ, van Wezel-Meijler G. Neonatal cranial ultrasonography: how to optimize its performance. Early Hum Dev. 2009;85:93–9. doi:10.1016/j.earlhumdev.2008.11.008.

van Wezel-Meijler G, Steggerda SJ, Leijser LM. Cranial ultrasonography in neonates: role and limitations. Semin Perinatol. 2010;34:28–38. doi:10.1053/j.semperi.2009.10.002.

Chapter 2
How to Perform a Neonatal Head Ultrasonography Study

For an informative, diagnostic ultrasonography (US) study of the neonatal brain, a modern, technologically advanced, US unit is essential. Various transducers including vector, curved array, and linear probes capable of scanning at multiple megahertz (MHz) settings should be provided and able to scan at a minimum of 15 MHz in order to reach the optimal tissue quality. Imaging algorithms should be optimized for the preterm (PT) and term (FT) neonatal brains. This "tuning" of the algorithms in cooperation with the manufacturer's technical representative can dramatically improve resolution, contrast, and detection of pathology and can provide a "high-end" approach for each case.

The study should begin with gray-scale anatomical images accessed through the anterior fontanel (AF) covering the entire brain in coronal (Fig. 2.1) and sagittal (Fig. 2.2) planes. In addition, mastoid fontanel (MF) (Fig. 2.3), posterior fontanel (PF) (Figs. 2.4, 2.5 and 2.6), and suboccipital views through the foramen magnum should be included for a better exploration of the contents of the posterior fossa. Depending on the probe, 3-D data sets may be acquired that allow secondary multiplanar reconstructions which match the more typical CT and MRI imaging planes. Imaging should always take advantage of optimization of all selectable imaging settings including correct depth penetration, gain, number of foci, etc. Moreover, the chosen US probe should have a

© Springer International Publishing Switzerland 2016
A. Poretti, T.A.G.M. Huisman (eds.), *Neonatal Head and Spine Ultrasonography*, DOI 10.1007/978-3-319-14568-6_2

footprint that matches the size of the acoustic window, be positioned in the center of the fontanel and maintain good contact with the scalp through the use of appropriate amount of US gel (Daneman et al. 2006; Grant and White 1986; Steggerda et al. 2009; van Wezel-Meijler et al. 2010). Depending on the pathology encountered, more detailed assessment of lesions located along the convexity of the cerebral hemispheres may require additional scanning with higher frequency probes and oblique, off-center probe positioning (Fig. 2.7) (Correa et al. 2004; Di Salvo 2001; Enriquez et al. 2006; Leijser et al. 2006; Steggerda et al. 2009).

In addition to the gray-scale anatomical imaging, the resistive index (RI) of the intracranial vasculature can be sampled using Doppler US along an anterior branch of the circle of Willis, usually one of the anterior cerebral arteries (ACA) (Figs. 2.8 and 2.9). The RI value is calculated as the ratio between the maximal end-diastolic and end-systolic flow velocities (Peak Systolic Velocity-Minimum Diastolic Velocity/ Peak Systolic Velocity). For FT neonates, the normal RI is 0.65–0.75, while PT infants have a slightly higher RI value (0.77–0.8) (Fig. 2.10) (Huisman et al. 2010; Zamora et al. 2014). The RI values are best measured at the beginning of the study through the AF without and then with gentle pressure being applied with the transducer. A large variability in the RI values acquired with and without pressure may indicate impaired intracranial autoregulation. Subsequently, the superior sagittal sinus is sampled for patency and flow direction.

To date, there is no internationally adopted standard for optimal timing and frequency of neonatal head US. Each institution uses its own protocol currently (Horsch et al. 2010; Leijser et al. 2006; Nwafor-Anene et al. 2003; Steggerda et al. 2009; van Wezel-Meijler et al. 2010). The frequency of head US examinations should be intensified if there is a sudden deterioration in infant's clinical state: for example, sepsis, necrotizing enterocolitis, episodes of apnea and/or bradycardia, unexplained decrease in hemoglobin level, new onset of neurological symptoms or ventricular dilatation. Scanning is also advised before and after major surgery (van Wezel-Meijler et al. 2010).

Finally, communication between neonatologists/pediatricians taking care of the baby and pediatric radiologists about the symptoms and clinical findings of newborn is essential to best investigate the clinical suspicions, make the correct diagnosis, and avoid misdiagnoses.

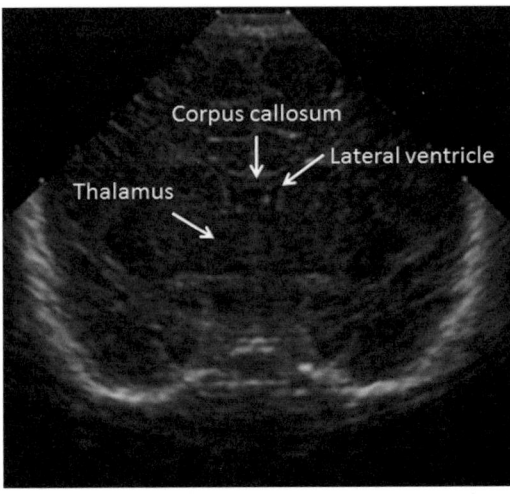

Fig. 2.1. Anterior fontanelle approach: coronal view. This technique is especially important to evaluate the lateral ventricles and choroid plexus. The corpus callosum appears above the cavum septum pellucidum. Caudate nuclei, putamen and globus pallidus, thalami, bilateral temporal lobes, uncus, hippocampi, and Sylvian fissures can be evaluated. The foramen of Monro, brainstem, and posterior fossa structures are also seen.

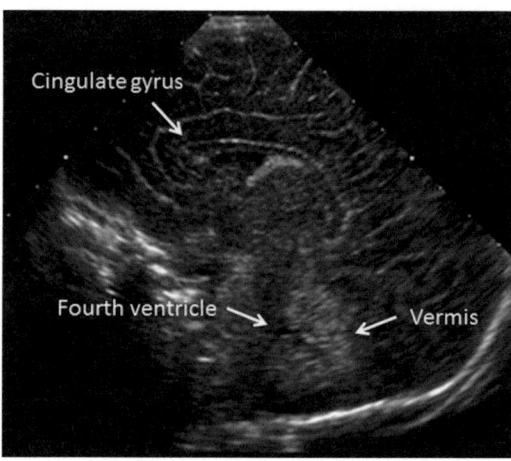

FIG. 2.2. Anterior fontanelle approach: midline sagittal view. The cerebellar vermis appears as an echogenic image in the posterior fossa. The fourth ventricle is placed in front of the vermis, the cisterna magna is placed below the cerebellar vermis and appears hypoechogenic. The corpus callosum is seen as a curve from anterior to posterior, cingulate gyrus appears above and parallel to it.

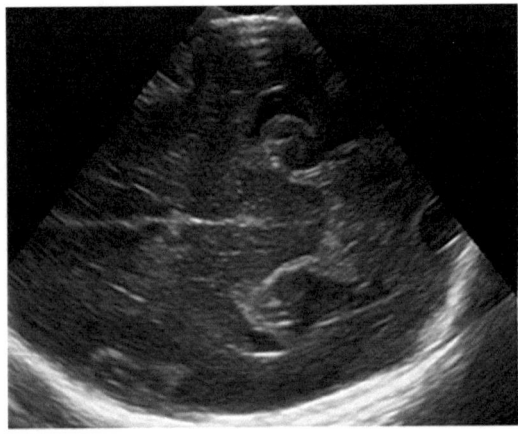

FIG. 2.3. Transmastoid approach: axial image. This technique allows to study the anatomy of the posterior fossa in more detail.

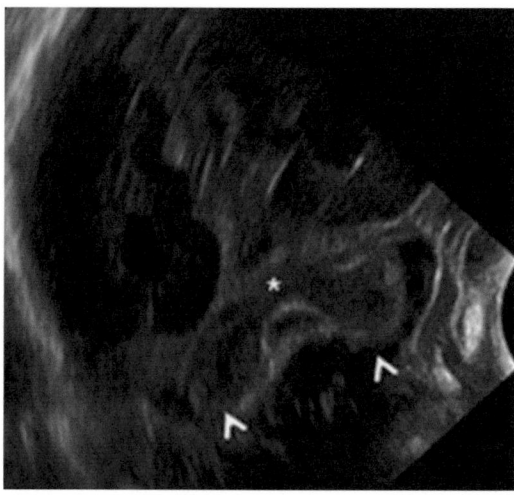

FIG. 2.4. Posterior fontanel approach: coronal image. This technique allows to study the anatomy of the posterior fossa in more detail and shows the craniocervical junction, cerebellar hemispheres (*arrowheads*), and cerebellar vermis (*asterix*) in high detail.

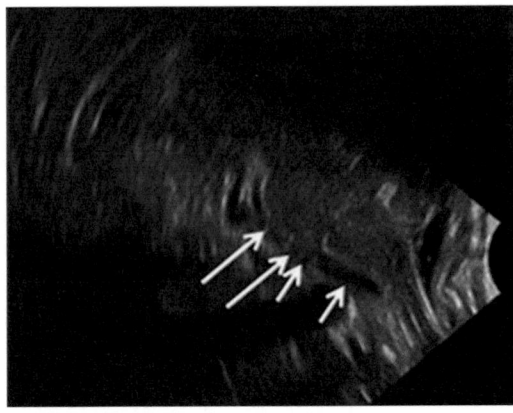

FIG. 2.5. Posterior fontanel approach: sagittal image. This technique allows to study the anatomy of the posterior fossa in more detail and shows the pons (*long arrows*) and remaining brainstem (*short arrows*) in high detail.

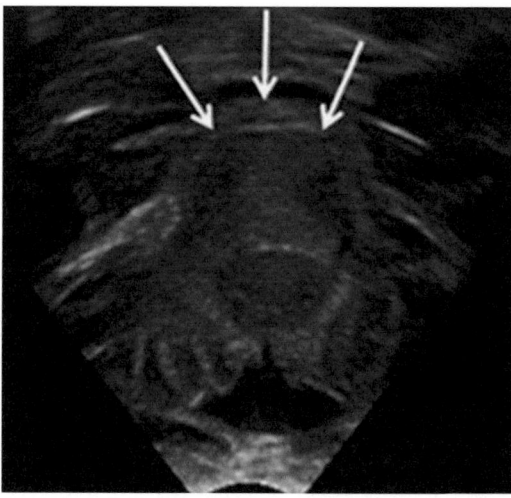

Fig. 2.6. Posterior fontanel approach: axial image. This technique allows to study the anatomy of the posterior fossa in more detail and shows the pons (*long arrows*) in high detail.

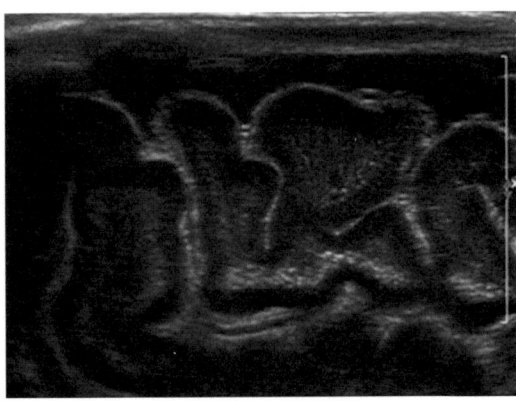

FIG. 2.7. High-resolution, high-frequency linear transducers allow to study the anatomy of the brain surface in high detail. This sagittal head ultrasound image has been acquired through the anterior fontanelle. The subarachnoid space is filled with clear, hypoechogenic CSF, the pia mater is seen as a hyperechogenic thin layer following the contour of the brain gyri, extending into the brain sulci. The cerebral cortex is slightly hypoechogenic in contrast to the mildly hyperechogenic subcortical white matter. The stripes within the WM represent the acoustic reflections of the intramedullary vessels.

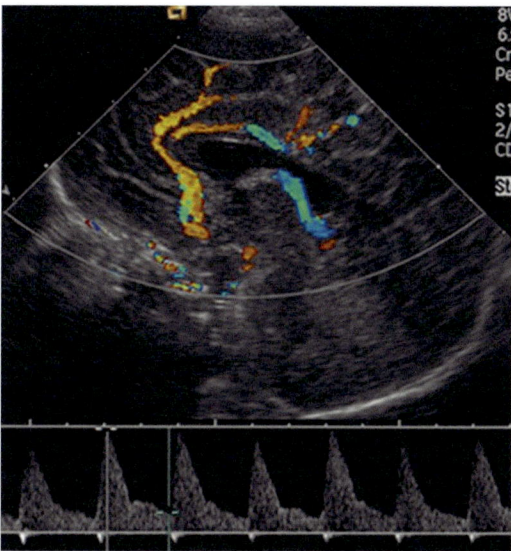

FIG. 2.8. Sagittal color-coded Doppler ultrasound evaluation of the circle of Willis in a normal term infant. *Red* coding indicates flow toward the location of the ultrasound probe, *blue* relates to flow away from the ultrasound probe. In addition, the flow profile over the cardiac cycle is shown with a steep increase of the cerebral blood flow velocity in the systole and a slower, but positive blood flow velocity during diastole.

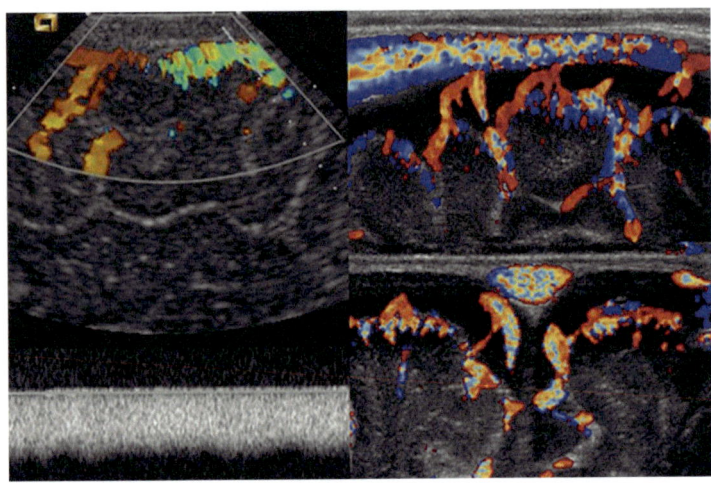

FIG. 2.9. Sagittal and coronal sampling of the superior sagittal sinus including adjacent draining bridging veins. The superior sagittal sinus is lined by the mildly hyperechogenic dura. Multiple veins are noted to cross the subdural space before draining into the superior sagittal sinus. Steady flow with minimal modulation is noted on the flow profile confirming patency of the superior sagittal sinus and normal flow direction.

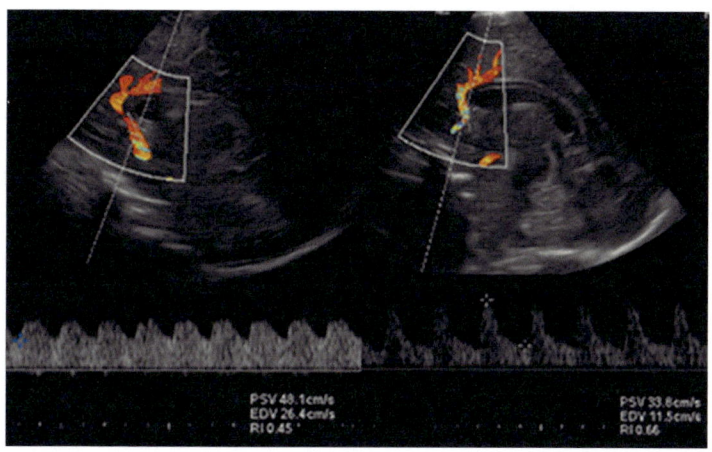

FIG. 2.10. Flow profile sampled from a branch of the anterior circulation through the anterior fontanelle. An elevated end diastolic velocity with resultant lowered RI value of 0.45 is seen in the first neonate with brain edema versus a RI value of 0.66 in the second healthy neonate. A lowered RI value may be seen in a variety of cerebral pathologies including inflammation, hypoxic-ischemic injury which impairs brain autoregulation.

References

Correa F, Enriquez G, Rossello J, Lucaya J, Piqueras J, Aso C, et al. Posterior fontanelle sonography: an acoustic window into the neonatal brain. AJNR Am J Neuroradiol. 2004;25:1274–82.

Daneman A, Epelman M, Blaser S, Jarrin JR. Imaging of the brain in full-term neonates: does sonography still play a role? Pediatr Radiol. 2006;36:636–46.

Di Salvo DN. A new view of the neonatal brain: clinical utility of supplemental neurologic US imaging windows. Radiographics. 2001;21:943–55.

Enriquez G, Correa F, Aso C, Carreño JC, Gonzalez R, Padilla NF, Vazquez E. Mastoid fontanelle approach for sonographic imaging of the neonatal brain. Pediatr Radiol. 2006;36:532–40.

Grant EG, White EM. Pediatric neurosonography. J Child Neurol. 1986;1:319–37.

Horsch S, Kutz P, Roll C. Late germinal matrix hemorrhage-like lesions in very preterm infants. J Child Neurol. 2010;25:809–14. doi:10.1177/0883073809346849.

Huisman TA, Singhi S, Pinto PS. Non-invasive imaging of intracranial pediatric vascular lesions. Childs Nerv Syst. 2010;26:1275–95. doi:10.1007/s00381-010-1203-1.

Leijser LM, de Vries LS, Cowan FM. Using cerebral ultrasound effectively in the newborn infant. Early Hum Dev. 2006;82:827–35.

Nwafor-Anene VN, DeCristofaro JD, Baumgart S. Serial head ultrasound studies in preterm infants: how many normal studies does one infant need to exclude significant abnormalities? J Perinatol. 2003;23:104–10.

Steggerda SJ, Leijser LM, Walther FJ, van Wezel-Meijler G. Neonatal cranial ultrasonography: how to optimize its performance. Early Hum Dev. 2009;85:93–9. doi:10.1016/j.earlhumdev.2008.11.008.

van Wezel-Meijler G, Steggerda SJ, Leijser LM. Cranial ultrasonography in neonates: role and limitations. Semin Perinatol. 2010;34:28–38. doi:10.1053/j.semperi.2009.10.002.

Zamora C, Tekes A, Alqahtani E, Kalayci OT, Northington F, Huisman TA. Variability of resistive indices in the anterior cerebral artery during fontanel compression in preterm and term neonates measured by transcranial duplex sonography. J Perinatol. 2014;34:306–10. doi:10.1038/jp.2014.11.

Chapter 3
Normal Head Ultrasound in the Preterm and Term Newborn

The neonatal brain becomes increasingly sulcated/convoluted during development. The sulcation pattern in preterm neonates born before 24 weeks of gestation is characterized only by the Sylvian fissure, while the brain surface is otherwise smooth mimicking a lissencephalic brain (Figs. 3.1 and 3.2). At 24 weeks of gestation, the parieto-occipital fissure is seen. This is followed by the appearance of the cingulate gyrus at about 28 weeks of gestation with additional branching occurring into full term (Figs. 3.3, 3.4 and 3.5) (North and Lowe 2009; Rumack et al. 2005).

Healthy preterm and occasionally term neonates usually show persistent fetal fluid-filled spaces such as the cavum septum pellucidum (Fig. 3.1), cavum Vergae, and cavum veli interpositi. Commonly, these spaces start to close around the sixth month of gestation and in about 85 % of infants are completely closed by 3–6 months of postnatal age (Epelman et al. 2006; Needelman et al. 2007). The cavum septum pellucidum is a midline fluid-filled space located anteriorly and between the frontal horns of the lateral ventricles, while the cavum veli interpositi is located further posteriorly as a separate fluid-filled space found in the pineal region.

Asymmetrical size of the lateral ventricles is a common finding in neonates and occurs in about 20–40 % of preterm and term newborns (Middleton et al. 2009). This may appear as a discrepancy between the frontal and occipital horn size

© Springer International Publishing Switzerland 2016   19
A. Poretti, T.A.G.M. Huisman (eds.), *Neonatal Head and Spine Ultrasonography*, DOI 10.1007/978-3-319-14568-6_3

or as variations in sizes of the left and right ventricles. The left ventricle is most commonly the bigger of the two with sizes varying depending on patient position (Enriquez et al. 2006).

The choroid plexus is located along the roof of the third ventricle and extends through the foramen of Monro into the lateral ventricles (North and Lowe 2009). It does not extend into the frontal or occipital horns, so hyperechoic material in these areas suggests pathology (Fig. 3.6). Choroid plexus morphology, however, is variable and should not be confused with hemorrhage. This is especially true for the posterior lateral ventricles and ventricular atria where lobular and bulbous choroid is commonly seen. In preterm neonates, the choroid plexus has a more abundant appearance due to the smaller cerebral mantle.

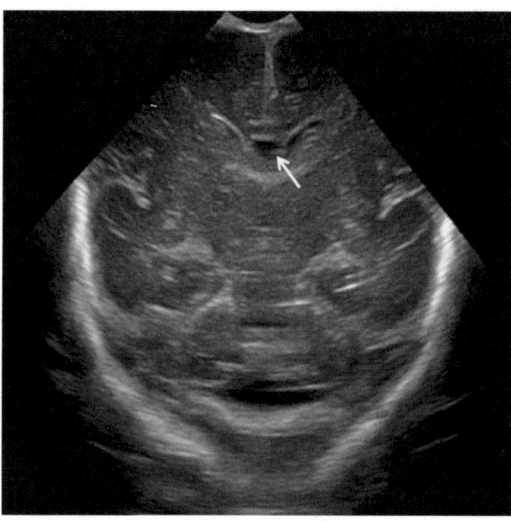

FIG. 3.1. Coronal image through the anterior fontanelle of a 10-day-old preterm neonate born at 25 weeks of gestation. The brain surface is smooth, a cavum septum pellucidum (*arrow*) is seen, and the lateral ventricles are slightly prominent. All these findings are related to prematurity and consequently normal for gestational age. The interface between cortex and subcortical white matter is ill-defined.

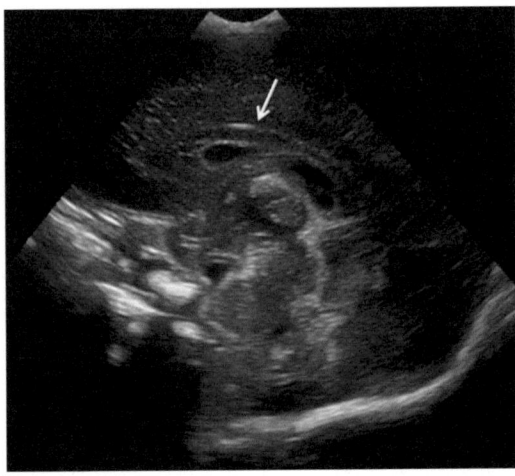

Fig. 3.2. Midsagittal image through the anterior fontanelle of a 10-day-old preterm neonate born at 25 weeks of gestation. The brain surface is smooth. The corpus callosum (*arrow*) is easily seen. The quadrigeminal plate is outlined by the hyperechogenic supravermian cistern. The vermis appears hyperechogenic, the fourth ventricle is filled with hypoechogenic cerebrospinal fluid.

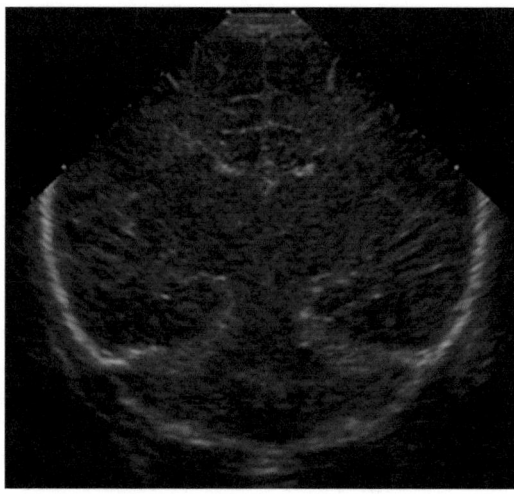

FIG. 3.3. Coronal image through the anterior fontanelle of a term neonate born at 38 weeks of gestation. The gray–white matter differentiation and maturation of the gyration and sulcation are nicely demonstrated.

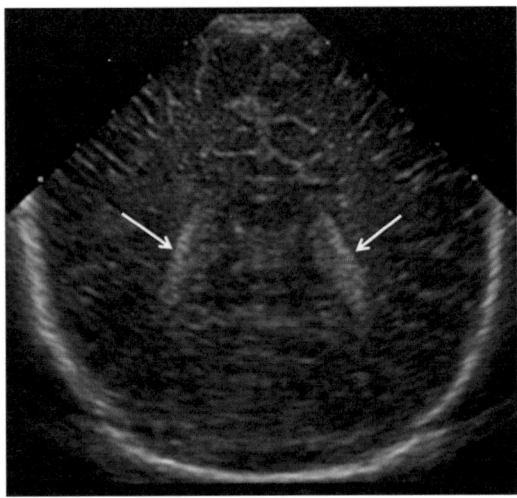

Fig. 3.4. Coronal image through the anterior fontanelle (posterior image compared to Fig. 3.2) of a term neonate born at 38 weeks of gestation. The lateral ventricles and choroid plexus (*arrows*) are better evaluated in these slices.

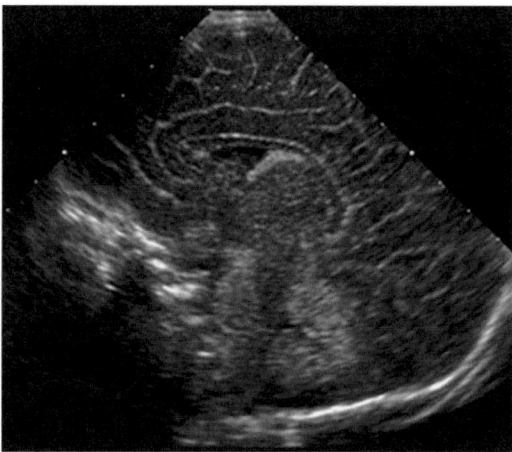

FIG. 3.5. Midsagittal image through the anterior fontanelle of a term neonate born at 38 weeks of gestation. The cerebellar vermis appears as an echogenic image in the posterior fossa. The fourth ventricle is placed in front of the vermis, the cisterna magna is placed below the cerebellar vermis and appears hypoechogenic. The corpus callosum is seen as a curve from anterior to posterior, cingulate gyrus appears above and parallel to it.

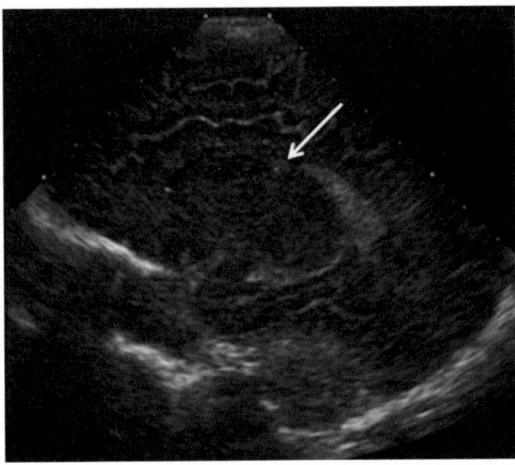

Fig. 3.6. Parasagittal image through the anterior fontanelle of a term neonate born at 38 weeks of gestation. The caudate nucleus is seen below the lateral ventricle, while the thalamus is located behind and below the caudate nucleus. The lateral ventricle is filled with choroid plexus. This view is the best view to evaluate the caudothalamic groove (*arrow*), an important landmark to evaluate germinal matrix hemorrhage.

References

Enriquez G, Correa F, Aso C, Carreño JC, Gonzalez R, Padilla NF, Vazquez E. Mastoid fontanelle approach for sonographic imaging of the neonatal brain. Pediatr Radiol. 2006;36:532–40.

Epelman M, Daneman A, Blaser SI, Ortiz-Neira C, Konen O, Jarrín J, Navarro OM. Differential diagnosis of intracranial cystic lesions at head US: correlation with CT and MR imaging. Radiographics. 2006;26:173–96.

Middleton WD, Kurtz AB, Hertzbert BS. Ultrasound: the requisites. St. Louis: Mosby; 2009.

Needelman H, Schroeder B, Sweeney M, Schmidt J, Bodensteiner JB, Schaefer GB. Postterm closure of the cavum septi pellucidi and developmental outcome in premature infants. J Child Neurol. 2007;22:314–6.

North K, Lowe L. Modern head ultrasound: normal anatomy, variants, and pitfalls that may simulate disease. Ultrasound Clin. 2009;4:497–512.

Rumack C, Wilson S, Charboneau J. Diagnostic ultrasound. St. Louis: Mosby; 2005.

Chapter 4
Seizures

Seizures are a common manifestation of a variety of neurological diseases in newborns (Girard and Raybaud 2011; Nagarajan et al. 2012; Plouin and Kaminska 2013; Vasudevan and Levene 2013). In neonates, five different clinical seizure patterns occur: subtle, multifocal clonic, focal clonic, tonic, and myoclonic (Abend and Wusthoff 2012). In contrast to older children, tonic–clonic seizures are extremely rare in newborns. Most cases of neonatal seizures are symptomatic with associated causal and risk factors, while few neonatal seizures are idiopathic (2–5 %). The most common etiologies of neonatal seizures include hypoxic-ischemic injury (Gillam-Krakauer and Carter 2012), cerebrovascular disorders such as arterial ischemic stroke and sinovenous thrombosis (Berfelo et al. 2010; Govaert et al. 2009), intracranial hemorrhages, acquired metabolic disorders such as hypoglycemia and hypocalcemia (Gataullina et al. 2015), infections including bacterial meningitis, viral meningoencephalitis (e.g., by herpes simplex), and congenital infections (Kimberlin and Whitley 2005; Mustonen et al. 2003), brain malformations, neurometabolic disorders such as urea cycle defects, mitochondrial disorders, and peroxisomal disorders (Van Hove and Lohr 2011), and maternal drug intoxication or neonatal drug withdrawal. It is important to identify neonatal seizures and their underlying cause as soon as possible to initiate an appropriate therapy and avoid further brain damages.

© Springer International Publishing Switzerland 2016
A. Poretti, T.A.G.M. Huisman (eds.), *Neonatal Head and Spine Ultrasonography*, DOI 10.1007/978-3-319-14568-6_4

High-quality neonatal head ultrasound may provide helpful information to detect or exclude various etiologies of neonatal seizures. In most cases, head ultrasonography allows to exclude lesions that require immediate treatment or neurosurgical intervention.

Differential Diagnosis of Brain Abnormalities Associated with Neonatal Seizures That May Be Detected by Neonatal Head Ultrasonography

– Hypoxic-ischemic encephalopathy (see Chap. 5)
– Arterial ischemic stroke
– Bacterial meningitis (see Chap. 5)
– Viral meningoencephalitis such as herpesvirus infection
– Congenital infection, e.g., by cytomegalovirus
– Intracranial hemorrhage
– Brain malformation such as lissencephaly, heterotopia, polymicrogyria, and holoprosencephaly
– Neurometabolic disorders such as urea cycle disorders, peroxisomal disorders, and mitochondrial disorders

Arterial Ischemic Stroke (Figs. 4.1 and 4.2)

At 22 days of life, a full-term male infant with Tetralogy of Fallot developed non-suppressible myoclonic jerking of the right upper extremity.

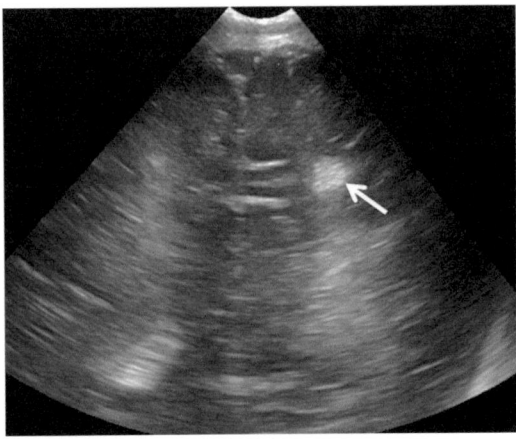

FIG. 4.1. Coronal image obtained through the anterior fontanelle of a 22-day-old term neonate with Tetralogy of Fallot shows hyperechogenic ischemic focus in left parietal region due to continuous ischemia.

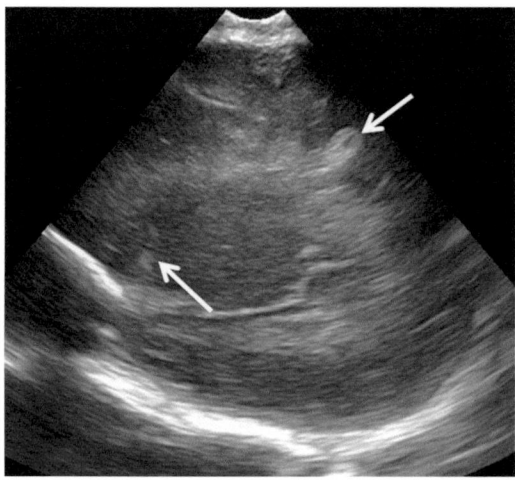

Fig. 4.2. Coronal image obtained through the anterior fontanelle of a 22-day-old term neonate with Tetralogy of Fallot reveals hyper-echogenic ischemic foci in left parietal and right temporal regions due to continuous ischemia.

Herpes Encephalitis (Figs. 4.3, 4.4, and 4.5)

A term newborn developed fever, lethargy, hypotonia, and clonic seizures at day of life 20. A lumbar puncture showed a lymphocytic pleocytosis.

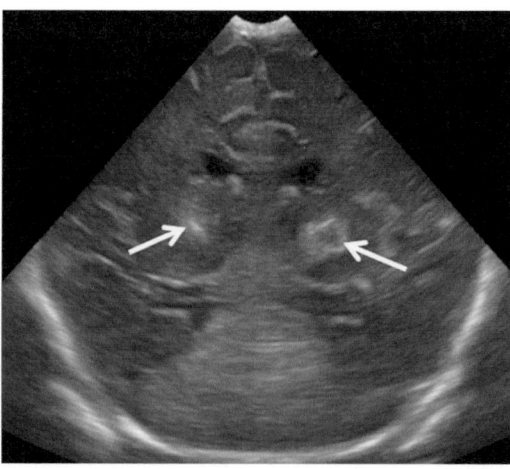

FIG. 4.3. Coronal image obtained through the anterior fontanelle of a 20-day-old term neonate with herpes simplex meningoencephalitis shows bilateral hyperechogenicity (*arrows*) of thalami left greater than right compatible with secondary ischemia and hemorrhagic conversion.

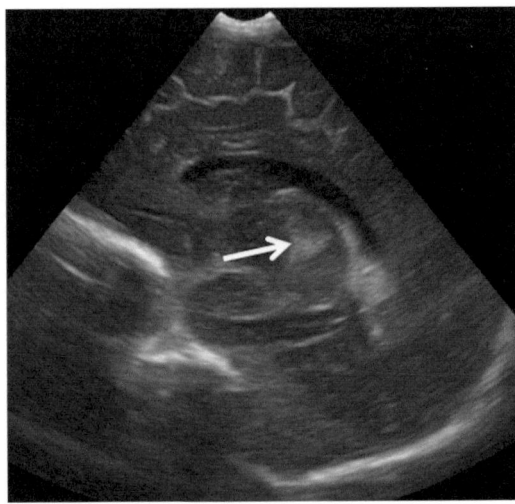

FIG. 4.4. Right parasagittal image obtained through the anterior fontanelle of a 20-day-old term neonate with herpes simplex meningoencephalitis reveals right-sided hyperechogenicity (*arrow*) of thalamus compatible with secondary ischemia and hemorrhagic conversion.

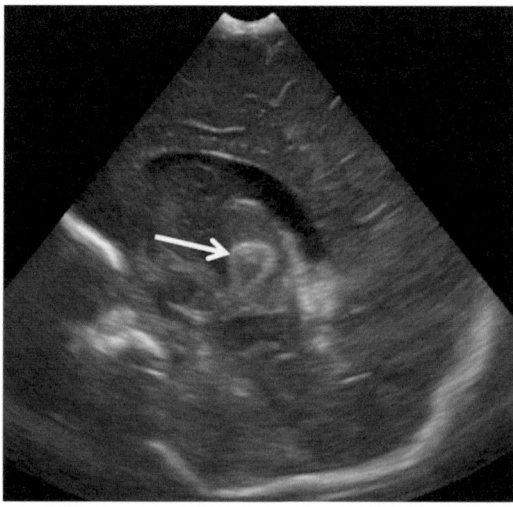

Fig. 4.5. Left parasagittal image obtained through the anterior fontanelle of a 20-day-old term neonate with herpes simplex meningoencephalitis shows left-sided hyperechogenicity (*arrow*) of thalamus compatible with secondary ischemia and hemorrhagic conversion.

Congenital Cytomegalovirus Infection (Figs. 4.6, 4.7, 4.8, and 4.9)

A full-term infant was prenatally diagnosed with intrauterine growth restriction. At birth, the infant was symmetrically small-for-gestational-age, had hepatosplenomegaly and diffuse, scattered purpura. Further work-up revealed bilateral chorioretinitis, optic atrophy, and failure of his hearing screening bilaterally. Labs showed hyperbilirubinemia, thrombocytopenia, and anemia.

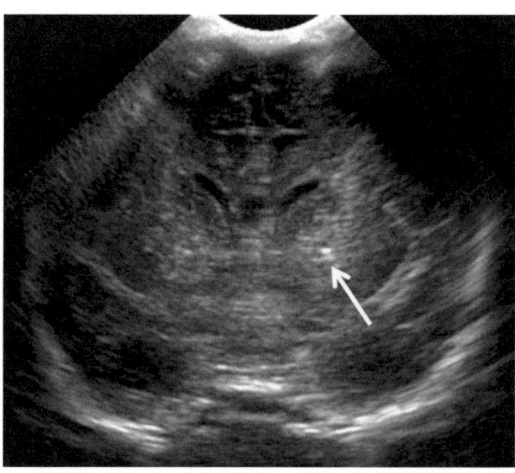

FIG. 4.6. Coronal image obtained through the anterior fontanelle of a term neonate with history of congenital cytomegalovirus infection shows multiple hyperechogenic foci suggestive of calcifications (*arrow*).

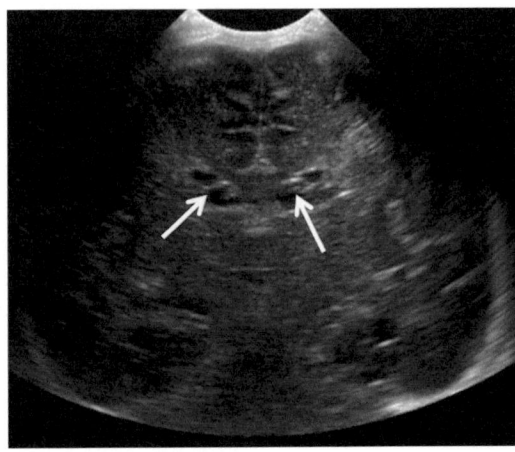

FIG. 4.7. Coronal image obtained through the anterior fontanelle of a term neonate with history of congenital cytomegalovirus infection reveals well-circumscribed intraventricular cysts bilaterally as usually seen in congenital infections (*arrow*).

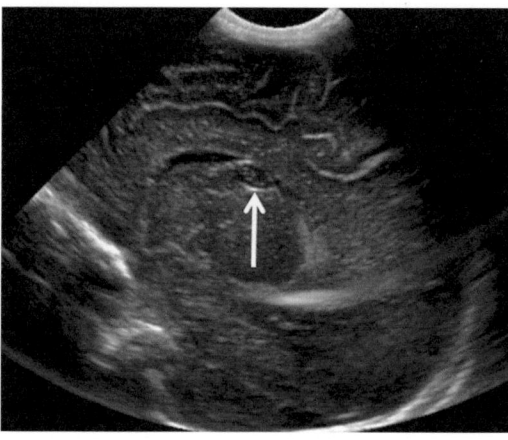

FIG. 4.8. Right parasagittal image obtained through the anterior fontanelle of a term neonate with history of congenital cytomegalovirus infection shows a well-circumscribed intraventricular cyst (*arrow*).

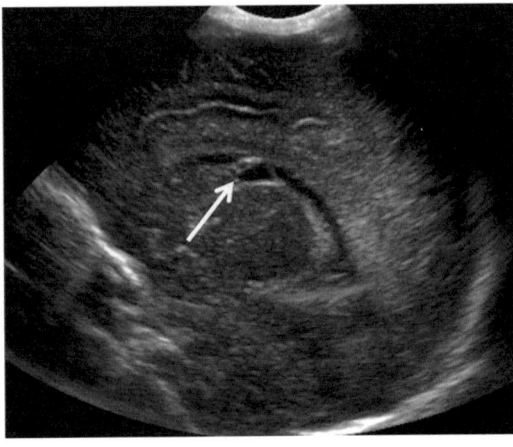

FIG. 4.9. Left parasagittal image obtained through the anterior fontanelle of a term neonate with history of congenital cytomegalovirus infection shows a well-circumscribed intraventricular cyst (*arrow*).

Intraventricular Hemorrhage with Periventricular Venous Infarction (Figs. 4.10 and 4.11)

A preterm neonate born at 30 weeks of gestation presented acute worsening of apneic events and clonic jerks of the left arm at day of life 7.

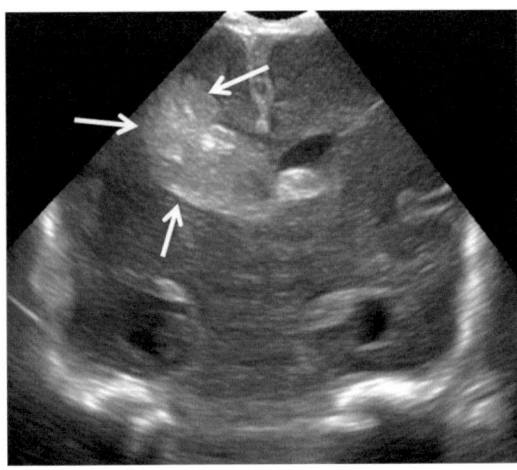

Fig. 4.10. Coronal image obtained through the anterior fontanelle of a 7-day-old neonate born at 30 weeks of gestation shows large bilateral germinal matrix hemorrhage with extensive right-sided periventricular venous infarction (*arrows*). Within the hyperechogenic white matter, multiple radiating hyperechogenic "stripes" are noted which relate to obstructed/thrombosed intramedullary veins.

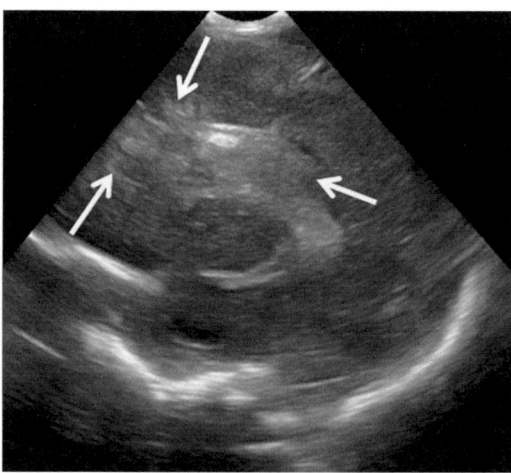

Fig. 4.11. Right parasaggital image obtained through the anterior fontanelle of a 7-day-old neonate born at 30 weeks of gestation reveals right-sided germinal matrix hemorrhage and periventricular venous infarction (*arrows*). Within the hyperechogenic white matter, multiple radiating hyperechogenic "stripes" are noted (*arrows*) which relate to obstructed/thrombosed intramedullary veins.

Periventricular Subependymal Heterotopia (Figs. 4.12 and 4.13)

A full-term infant was noted to have microcephaly and marked hypotonia at birth. She subsequently developed horizontal nystagmus, poor feeding, and jitteriness. On day seven of life, she has rhythmic jerking of her left arm, which is not suppressible.

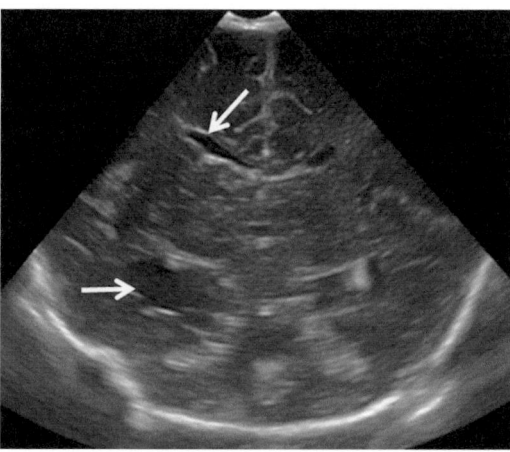

FIG. 4.12. Coronal image obtained through the anterior fontanelle of a 7-day-old term neonate with history of congenital ventriculomegaly shows enlargement of the lateral ventricles (*right>left*, *arrows*).

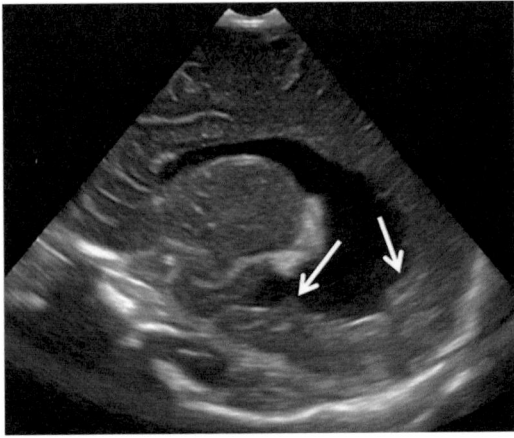

Fig. 4.13. Parasagittal image obtained through the anterior fontanelle of a 7-day-old term neonate with history of congenital ventriculomegaly reveals nodularity and irregular lining in the lateral ventricle wall (*arrow*), which may represent heterotopic gray matter.

References

Abend NS, Wusthoff CJ. Neonatal seizures and status epilepticus. J Clin Neurophysiol. 2012;29:441–8.

Berfelo FJ, Kersbergen KJ, van Ommen CH, Govaert P, van Straaten HL, Poll-The BT, van Wezel-Meijler G, Vermeulen RJ, Groenendaal F, de Vries LS, de Haan TR. Neonatal cerebral sinovenous thrombosis from symptom to outcome. Stroke. 2010;41:1382–8.

Gataullina S, Delonlay P, Lemaire E, Boddaert N, Bulteau C, Soufflet C, Laín GA, Nabbout R, Chiron C, Dulac O. Seizures and epilepsy in hypoglycemia caused by inborn errors of metabolism. Dev Med Child Neurol. 2015;57(2):194–9. doi:10.1111/dmcn.12574.

Gillam-Krakauer M, Carter BS. Neonatal hypoxia and seizures. Pediatr Rev. 2012;33:387–96.

Girard N, Raybaud C. Neonates with seizures: what to consider, how to image. Magn Reson Imaging Clin N Am. 2011;19:685–708.

Govaert P, Smith L, Dudink J. Diagnostic management of neonatal stroke. Semin Fetal Neonatal Med. 2009;14:323–8.

Kimberlin DW, Whitley RJ. Neonatal herpes: what have we learned. Semin Pediatr Infect Dis. 2005;16:7–16.

Mustonen K, Mustakangas P, Uotila L, Muir P, Koskiniemi M. Viral infections in neonates with seizures. J Perinat Med. 2003;31: 75–80.

Nagarajan L, Palumbo L, Ghosh S. Classification of clinical semiology in epileptic seizures in neonates. Eur J Paediatr Neurol. 2012;16: 118–25.

Plouin P, Kaminska A. Neonatal seizures. Handb Clin Neurol. 2013;111:467–76.

Van Hove JL, Lohr NJ. Metabolic and monogenic causes of seizures in neonates and young infants. Mol Genet Metab. 2011;104:214–30.

Vasudevan C, Levene M. Epidemiology and aetiology of neonatal seizures. Semin Fetal Neonatal Med. 2013;18:185–91.

Chapter 5
Encephalopathy

Neonatal encephalopathy refers to a neonatal neurological syndrome with clinical features consistent with a disorder of the brain. The most notable clinical features are depression of level of consciousness and seizures that are usually associated with respiratory depression, abnormalities of tone and power, and disturbances of cranial nerve function with impaired feeding (Volpe 2012). Hypoxic-ischemic injury is the main cause of neonatal encephalopathy (Chao et al. 2006; Epelman et al. 2012; Swarte et al. 2009). In hypoxic-ischemic injury, different patterns of injury have been described dependent on the gestational age of the neonate as well as duration and severity of hypoxia/ischemia (Volpe 2012):

1. Severe, prolonged hypoxic-ischemic injury typically involves the cerebral cortex, parasagittal subcortical/central white matter, deep gray matter nuclei (thalamus and basal ganglia, especially putamen), and brain stem (inferior colliculus and tegmentum).
2. Moderate, prolonged, and/or intermittent hypoxic-ischemic injury involves the cerebral cortex and parasagittal subcortical/central white matter, the deep gray matter nuclei (thalamus and basal ganglia, especially putamen), or, most commonly, both.
3. Severe, relatively brief hypoxic-ischemic injury involves the thalamus and basal ganglia, especially putamen, and brain stem (inferior colliculus and tegmentum).

© Springer International Publishing Switzerland 2016
A. Poretti, T.A.G.M. Huisman (eds.), *Neonatal Head and Spine Ultrasonography*, DOI 10.1007/978-3-319-14568-6_5

4. Mild/moderate, gradual/prolonged hypoxic-ischemic injury involves the periventricular/central cerebral white matter as the dominant lesion.

Hypoxic-ischemic injury, however, is not the only etiology of neonatal encephalopathy, which may be caused by a myriad of other disorders including intracranial hemorrhage (Owens 2005), hypoglycemia (Cakmakci et al. 2001), intracranial infection such as bacterial meningitis and viral encephalitis (Yikilmaz and Taylor 2008), severe hyperbilirubinemia (kernicterus) (Gkoltsiou et al. 2008), and neurometabolic disorders such as urea cycle disorders, maple syrup urine disease, sulfite oxidase deficiency, and non-ketotic hyperglycinemia (Leijser et al. 2007). The differentiation between the various etiologies of neonatal encephalopathy is mandatory in terms of therapy, prognosis, and family counseling regarding recurrence risk. High-quality neonatal head ultrasound enables accurate early visualization of different patterns of hypoxic-ischemic injury and detection of other etiologies of neonatal encephalopathy.

Differential Diagnosis of Brain Abnormalities Associated with Neonatal Encephalopathy That May Be Detected by Neonatal Head Ultrasonography

- Hypoxic-ischemic encephalopathy
- Intraventricular hemorrhage
- Intracranial, extraaxial hemorrhage
- Bacterial meningitis
- Viral meningoencephalitis (e.g., herpesvirus infection)
- Neurometabolic disorders (e.g., maple syrup urine disease)

Hypoxic-ischemic Injury (Figs. 5.1, 5.2, and 5.3)

A full-term infant was born via emergency C-section for prolonged fetal bradycardia in the setting of a placental abruption. His exam was notable for minimal spontaneous movement, poor respiratory effort, and hypotonia. His liver enzymes and creatinine were elevated. At around 8 h of life, lip smacking and bicycling movements of the extremities that could not be suppressed were noted.

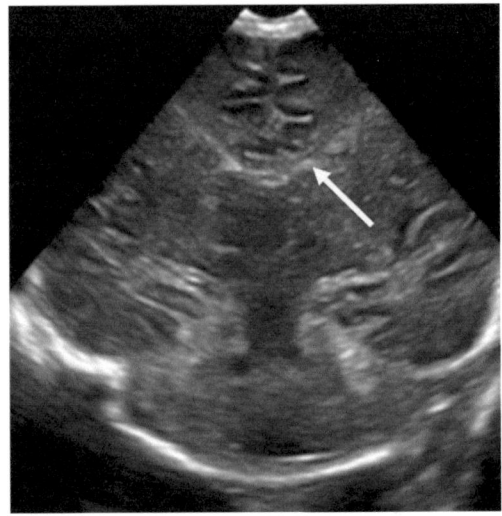

FIG. 5.1. Coronal image obtained through the anterior fontanelle of a term neonate with severe hypoxic-ischemic injury shows a white matter edema with hyperechogenicity of the white matter, increased cortico-medullary differentiation, and slit-like lateral ventricles (*arrow*).

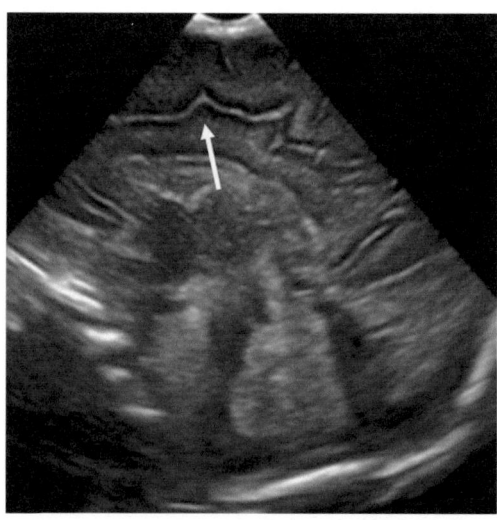

FIG. 5.2. Sagittal image obtained through the anterior fontanelle of a term neonate with severe hypoxic-ischemic injury reveals a white matter edema with hyperechogenicity of the white matter and increased cortico-medullary differentiation (*arrow*).

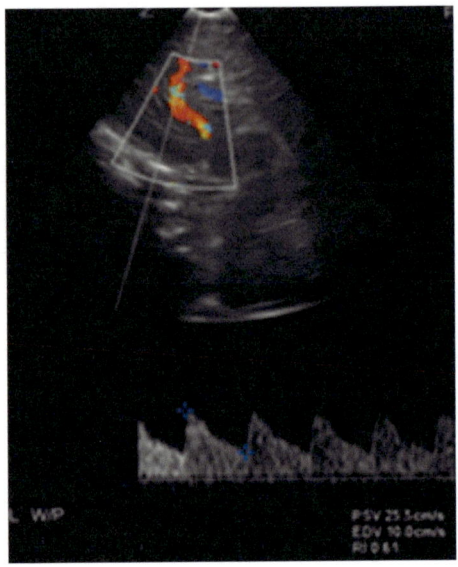

FIG. 5.3. Sagittal color-coded Doppler sonography evaluation of the circle of Willis of a term neonate with severe hypoxic-ischemic injury shows a low resistive index (RI) value sampled within a branch of the anterior circle of Willis (RI = 0.61). For term neonates, normal RI values range between 0.65 and 0.75, while preterm newborns have a slightly higher RI value (0.77–0.8).

Intraventricular Hemorrhage (Figs. 5.4 and 5.5)

A 5-day-old 28-week gestational age newborn has a sudden drop in her level of consciousness and increase in number of apneic and bradycardic events. On examination, she is noted to have decreased tone from baseline.

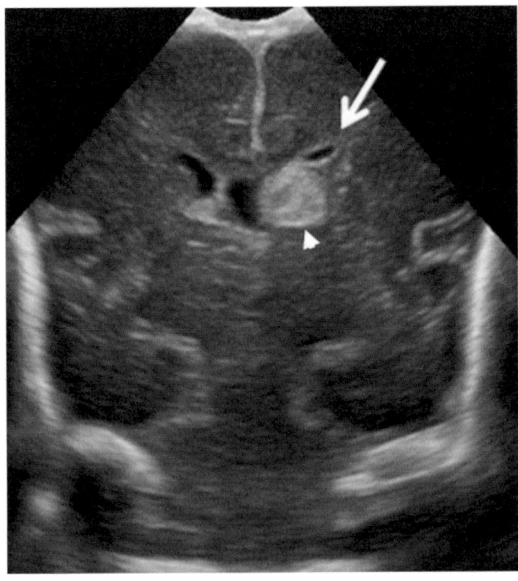

Fig. 5.4. Coronal image obtained through the anterior fontanelle of a 5-day-old 28-week gestational age newborn shows a medium-sized focal hyperechogenic hemorrhage in the left caudothalamic groove (*arrowhead*) next to a small hemorrhage on the *right*. The ependymal lining of the left lateral ventricle is mildly hyperechogenic (*arrow*) due to an inflammatory reaction secondary to intraventricular blood products as well as a mild venous stasis. The ventricles are normal in size. The findings are consistent of grade 2 germinal matrix hemorrhage.

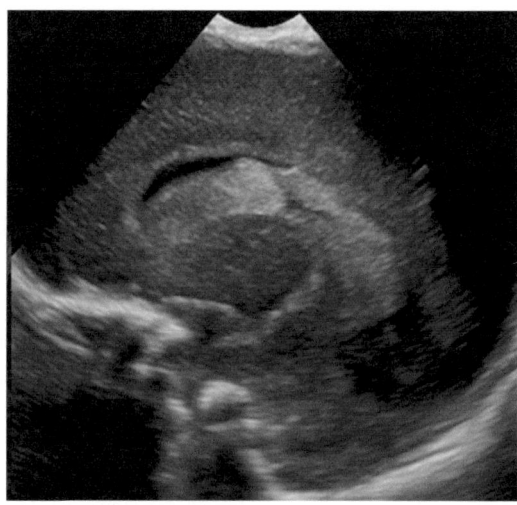

Fig. 5.5. Sagittal image obtained through the anterior fontanelle of a 5-day-old 28-week gestational age newborn reveals the intraventricular extension of the hemorrhage of a left-sided grade 2 germinal matrix hemorrhage.

Subdural Hematoma (Figs. 5.6, 5.7, and 5.8)

A full-term large-for-gestational-age infant was born to a diabetic mother via a difficult vaginal delivery that required forceps-assistance, resulting in a large cephalohematoma. He was transferred to the intensive care unit after developing cyanotic episodes, increased irritability, and hypoglycemia due to poor feeding.

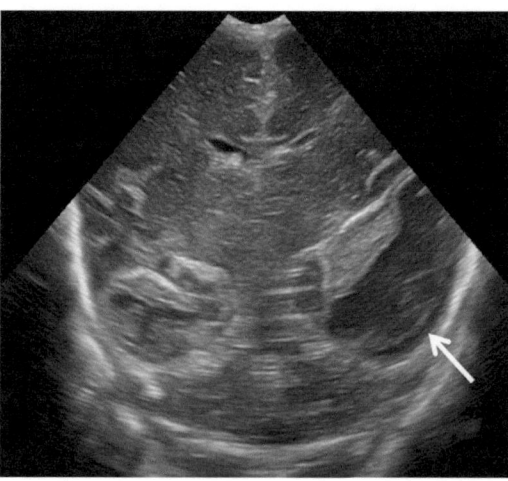

FIG. 5.6. Coronal image obtained through the anterior fontanelle of an 18-day-old term neonate shows bilateral subdural hemorrhages, *left* (*arrow*) greater than *right*. In addition, the left lateral ventricle is compressed and minimally cranially displaced due to the mass effect of hemorrhage.

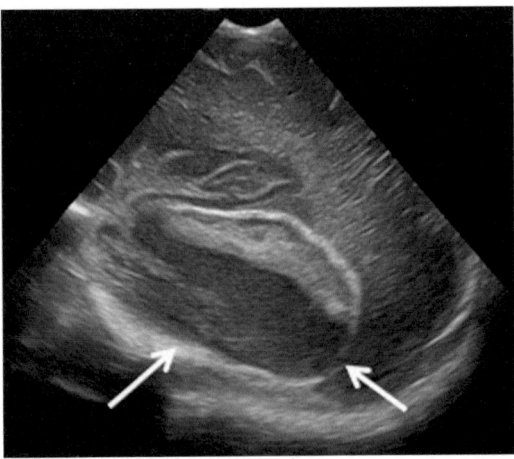

FIG. 5.7. Left parasagittal image obtained through the anterior fontanelle of an 18-day-old term neonate reveals a large subdural hemorrhage (*arrow*).

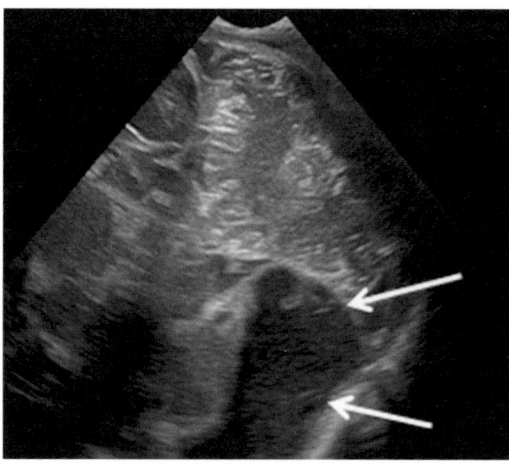

FIG. 5.8. Right transmastoid image of an 18-day-old term neonate shows bilateral subdural hemorrhages, *left (arrow)* greater than *right.*

Bacterial Meningitis (Figs. 5.9 and 5.10)

An infant was born at 32 weeks gestational age following prolonged rupture of membranes and maternal fever just prior to delivery. The infant developed hypotension, hypoglycemia, and increased irritability. Several hours later, the nurse noted tonic–clonic shaking of the right arm, which spread to the rest of his body. Labs showed a metabolic acidosis and elevated white blood cell count with an immature to total neutrophil ratio of 0.3. A lumbar puncture showed a neutrophilic pleocytosis with high protein and low glucose levels in the cerebral spinal fluid.

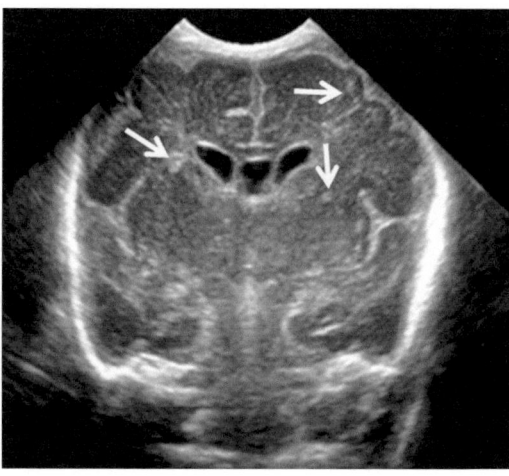

FIG. 5.9. Coronal image obtained through the anterior fontanelle of a 1-month-old preterm neonate born at 27 weeks of gestation with history of fungal sepsis and bacterial meningitis shows multiple rounded echogenic foci within the brain parenchyma bilaterally (*arrows*) concerning for micro-abscesses.

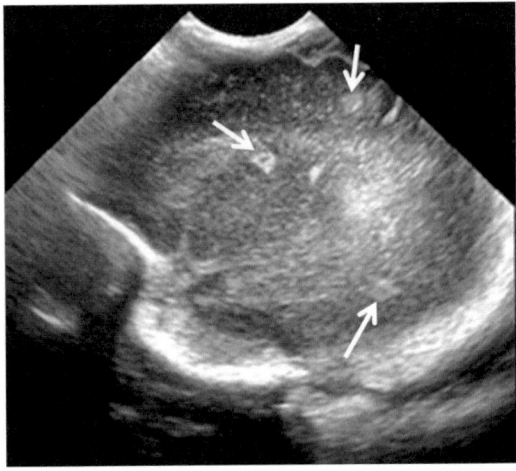

FIG. 5.10. Right parasagittal image obtained through the anterior fontanelle of a 1-month-old preterm neonate born at 27 weeks of gestation with history of fungal sepsis and bacterial meningitis shows multiple rounded echogenic foci within the brain parenchyma (*arrows*) concerning for micro-abscesses.

Herpes Encephalitis (Figs. 5.11, 5.12, and 5.13)

A preterm infant was born at 31 weeks gestational age to a mother with negative serologies via spontaneous vaginal delivery and was admitted to the NICU for prematurity. On day of life twelve, the infant developed lethargy, hypotonia, and clonic shaking. Following a fever to 39 °C, a lumbar puncture showed a lymphocytic pleocytosis with a mildly reduced CSF glucose.

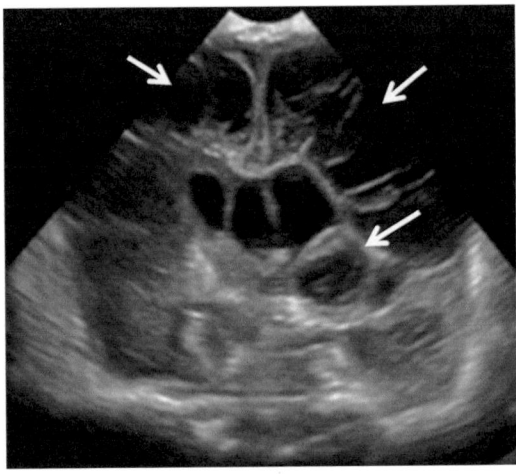

FIG. 5.11. Coronal image obtained through the anterior fontanelle of a 12-day-old preterm neonate born at 31 weeks of gestation with herpes simplex encephalitis shows heterogeneous cystic encephalomalacic changes (*arrows*) in the bilateral frontoparietal and left temporal lobes and left basal ganglia.

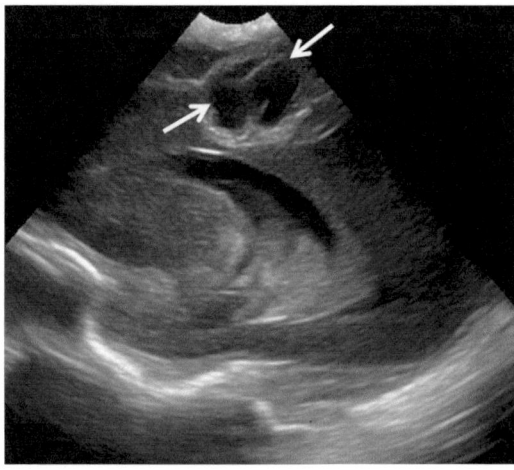

FIG. 5.12. Right parasagittal image obtained through the anterior fontanelle of a 12-day-old preterm neonate born at 31 weeks of gestation with herpes simplex encephalitis reveals heterogeneous cystic encephalomalacic changes (*arrow*) in the right frontoparietal lobe.

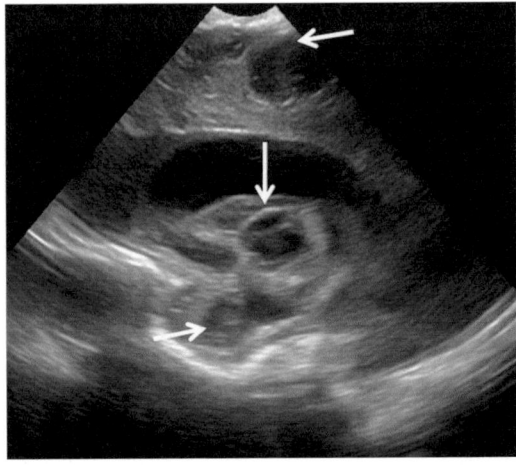

Fɪɢ. 5.13. Left parasagittal image obtained through the anterior fontanelle of a 12-day-old preterm neonate born at 31 weeks of gestation with herpes simplex encephalitis shows heterogeneous cystic encephalomalacic changes (*arrows*) in the left frontoparietal and temporal lobes and basal ganglia.

Maple Syrup Urine Disease (Figs. 5.14 and 5.15)

A 5-day-old full-term newborn develops feeding difficulties, a shrill cry, vomiting, and stupor followed by boxing and bicycling movements of the extremities. Clinical examination revealed variable muscle tone between flaccidity and spasticity. Plasma amino acid concentrations showed increased level of leucine, isoleucine, and valine.

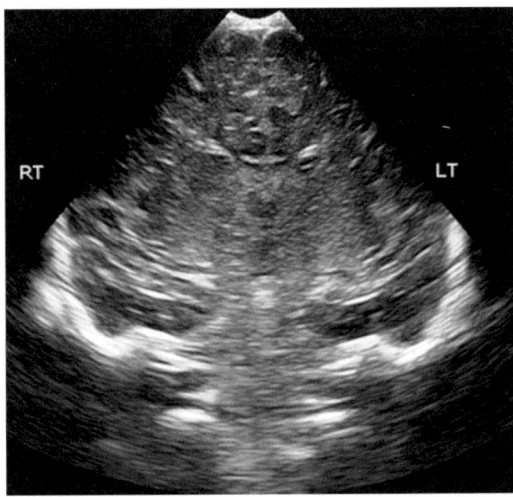

FIG. 5.14. Coronal image obtained through the anterior fontanelle of an 8-day-old term neonate with maple syrup urine disease shows diffuse hyperechogenicity of the white matter with slit-like ventricles, which is consistent with diffuse cerebral edema.

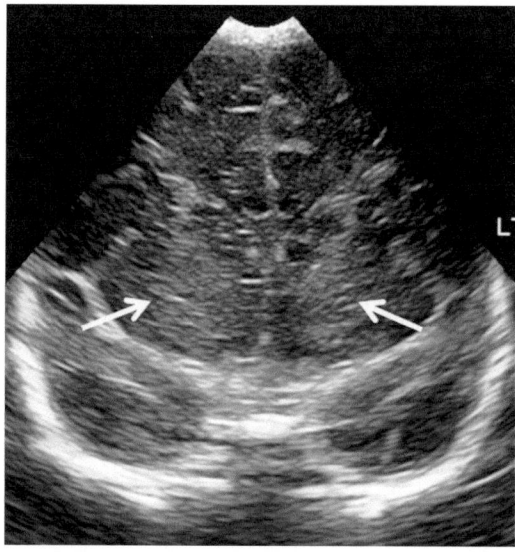

FIG. 5.15. Coronal image obtained through the anterior fontanelle of an 8-day-old term neonate with maple syrup urine disease reveals diffuse hyperechogenicity of the white matter with slit-like ventricles, which is consistent with diffuse cerebral edema. In addition, basal ganglia and thalami are slightly hyperechogenic (*arrows*) due to the intramyelinic edema.

References

Cakmakci H, Usal C, Karabay N, Kovanlikaya A. Transient neonatal hypoglycemia: cranial US and MRI findings. Eur Radiol. 2001; 11:2585–8.

Chao CP, Zaleski CG, Patton AC. Neonatal hypoxic-ischemic encephalopathy: multimodality imaging findings. Radiographics. 2006;26:S159–66.

Epelman M, Daneman A, Chauvin N, Hirsch W. Head Ultrasound and MR imaging in the evaluation of neonatal encephalopathy: competitive or complementary imaging studies? Magn Reson Imaging Clin N Am. 2012;20:93–115.

Gkoltsiou K, Tzoufi M, Counsell S, Rutherford M, Cowan F. Serial brain MRI and ultrasound findings: relation to gestational age, bilirubin level, neonatal neurologic status and neurodevelopmental outcome in infants at risk of kernicterus. Early Hum Dev. 2008;84: 829–38.

Leijser LM, de Vries LS, Rutherford MA, Manzur AY, Groenendaal F, de Koning TJ, van der Heide-Jalving M, Cowan FM. Cranial ultrasound in metabolic disorders presenting in the neonatal period: characteristic features and comparison with MR imaging. AJNR Am J Neuroradiol. 2007;28:1223–31.

Owens R. Intraventricular hemorrhage in the premature neonate. Neonatal Netw. 2005;24:55–571.

Swarte R, Lequin M, Cherian P, et al. Imaging patterns of brain injury in term-birth asphyxia. Acta Paediatr. 2009;98:586–92.

Volpe JJ. Neonatal encephalopathy: an inadequate term for hypoxic-ischemic encephalopathy. Ann Neurol. 2012;66:156–66.

Yikilmaz A, Taylor GA. Sonographic findings in bacterial meningitis in neonates and young infants. Pediatr Radiol. 2008;38:129–37.

Chapter 6
Muscular Hypotonia

Tone is defined as the resistance of muscle to stretch. Hypotonia refers to a reduced muscle tone and may be caused by injury of both the central and peripheral nervous system (Bodensteiner 2008; Lisi and Cohn 2011; Richer et al. 2001). Here we will focus on causes for neonatal muscular hypotonia secondary to injury of the central nervous system. Etiologies for neonatal muscular hypotonia due to injury of the central nervous system include hypoxic-ischemic encephalopathy, cerebellar hemorrhages, chromosomal disorders such as Prader–Willi syndrome, Down syndrome, and other trisomies, brain malformations such as lissencephaly and Joubert syndrome, neurometabolic disorders such as Zellweger syndrome, Smith–Lemli–Opitz syndrome, and congenital disorders of glycosylation (Leijser et al. 2007), and other genetic disorders such as Lowe syndrome. Neonatal head ultrasound provides helpful information in detecting brain abnormalities that may cause neonatal muscular hypotonia.

© Springer International Publishing Switzerland 2016   75
A. Poretti, T.A.G.M. Huisman (eds.), *Neonatal Head and Spine Ultrasonography*, DOI 10.1007/978-3-319-14568-6_6

Differential Diagnosis of Brain Abnormalities Associated with Muscular Hypotonia That May Be Detected by Neonatal Head Ultrasonography

– Hypoxic-ischemic encephalopathy (see Chap. 4)
– Cerebellar hemorrhage (see Chap. 8)
– Lissencephaly (see Chap. 4)
– Schizencephaly (see Chap. 9)
– Joubert syndrome

Joubert Syndrome (Figs. 6.1, 6.2, and 6.3)

A full-term infant with a history of cerebellar hypoplasia on prenatal ultrasound appeared hypotonic at birth and had to be intubated due to respiratory distress and apnea. He was also noted to have an additional fifth digit on his left hand.

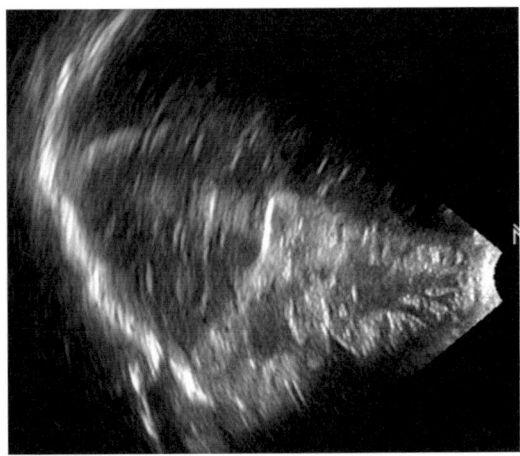

FIG. 6.I. Coronal image obtained through the anterior fontanel of a term neonate with Joubert syndrome, global hypotonia, and breathing abnormalities shows a moderate bilateral ventriculomegaly and hypoplasia of the cerebellar vermis

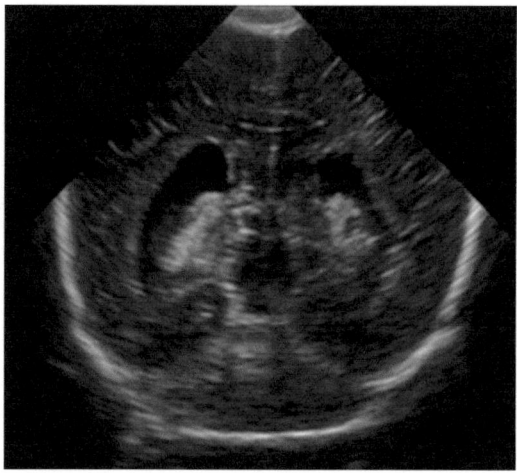

Fɪɢ. 6.2. Sagittal image obtained through the anterior fontanel of a term neonate with Joubert syndrome, global hypotonia, and breathing abnormalities reveals hypoplasia of the cerebellar vermis (*arrow*) with secondary dilatation of the fourth ventricle.

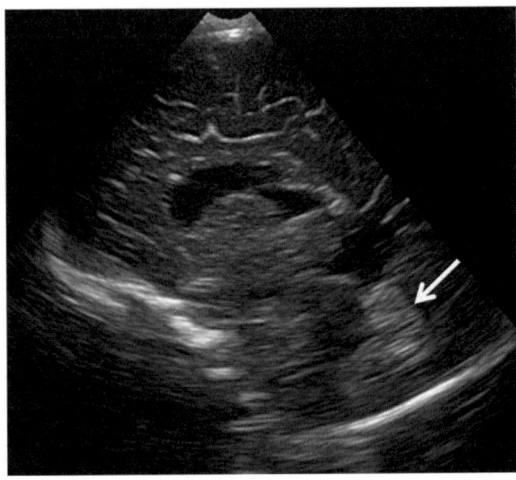

FIG. 6.3. Axial image obtained through the left mastoid of a term neonate with Joubert syndrome, global hypotonia, and breathing abnormalities shows hypoplasia of the cerebellar vermis (*arrow*) with secondary dilatation of the fourth ventricle.

References

Bodensteiner JB. The evaluation of the hypotonic infant. Semin Pediatr Neurol. 2008;15:10–20.

Leijser LM, de Vries LS, Rutherford MA, Manzur AY, Groenendaal F, de Koning TJ, van der Heide-Jalving M, Cowan FM. Cranial ultrasound in metabolic disorders presenting in the neonatal period: characteristic features and comparison with MR imaging. AJNR Am J Neuroradiol. 2007;28:1223–31.

Lisi EC, Cohn RD. Genetic evaluation of the pediatric patient with hypotonia: perspective from a hypotonia specialty clinic and review of the literature. Dev Med Child Neurol. 2011;53:586–99.

Richer LP, Shevell MI, Miller SP. Diagnostic profile of neonatal hypotonia: an 11-year study. Pediatr Neurol. 2001;25:32–7.

Chapter 7
Hemiparesis

Hemiparesis is defined as weakness involving one side of the body. In newborns, it usually appears as reduced spontaneous movement of one body side. Hemiparesis and hemiplegia, its most severe form, may be caused by injury of both the central and peripheral nervous system. Here we will focus on causes for neonatal hemiparesis and hemiplegia secondary to injury of the central nervous system. Etiologies for neonatal hemiparesis due to injury of the central nervous system include arterial ischemic stroke (Abels et al. 2006; Govaert 2009; van der Aa et al. 2014), unilateral intracranial hemorrhage (mostly involving the parietal or temporal lobes), unilateral periventricular venous infarction (de Vries et al. 2001; Dudink et al. 2008; Huisman 2005), and unilateral brain malformations such as hemimegalencephaly or unilateral migration disorders. Neonatal head ultrasound provides helpful information in detecting brain abnormalities that may cause neonatal hemiparesis or hemiplegia.

© Springer International Publishing Switzerland 2016   83
A. Poretti, T.A.G.M. Huisman (eds.), *Neonatal Head and Spine Ultrasonography*, DOI 10.1007/978-3-319-14568-6_7

Differential Diagnosis of Brain Abnormalities Associated with Hemiparesis/Hemiplegia That May Be Detected by Neonatal Head Ultrasonography

- Arterial ischemic stroke
- Unilateral intracranial hemorrhage
- Unilateral periventricular venous infarction
- Unilateral brain malformations such as hemimegalencephaly or unilateral migrational abnormalities

Arterial Ischemic Stroke (Figs. 7.1 and 7.2)

A full-term male infant was delivered after an episode of fetal bradycardia to a mother with intrapartum fever. At 14 h of life, he developed non-suppressible myoclonic jerking of the left upper extremity. A new cardiac murmur is appreciated on exam, and tetralogy of Fallot was diagnosed via echocardiogram.

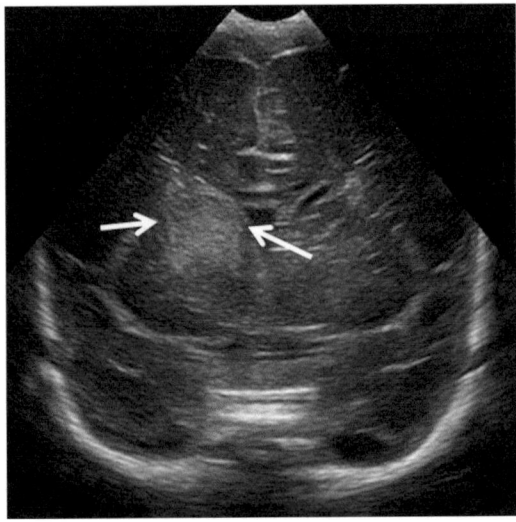

FIG. 7.1. Coronal image obtained through the anterior fontanelle of a 31-weeker preterm neonate at day of life 21 shows a focal hyperechogenic lesion (*arrows*) with mild mass effect within right basal ganglia. This lesion is concerning for an ischemic stroke. In addition, the adjacent anterior horn of the right lateral ventricle appears smaller than the contralateral side.

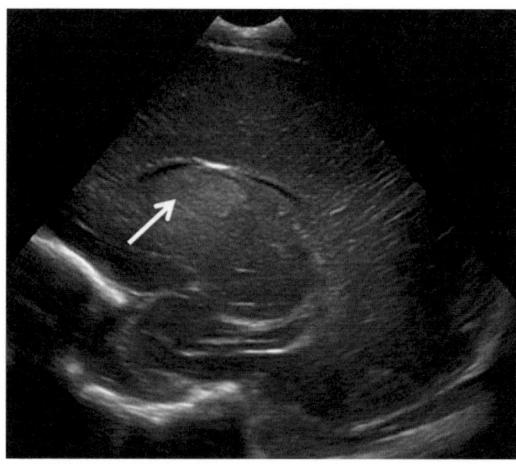

Fig. 7.2. Right parasagittal image obtained through the anterior fontanelle of a 31-weeker preterm neonate at day of life 21 reveals a focal hyperechogenic lesion (*arrow*) with mild mass effect within basal ganglia on the right side.

Intraventricular Hemorrhage (Figs. 7.3, 7.4, and 7.5)

A preterm neonate born at 32 weeks of gestation presented acute worsening of apneic events at day of life 6. Clinical evaluation revealed asymmetric muscle tone that was reduced on the left side.

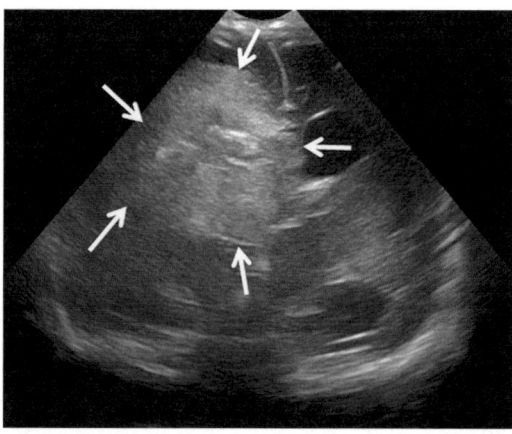

FIG. 7.3. Coronal image obtained through the anterior fontanelle of a 2-day-old preterm neonate born at 32 weeks of gestation shows a large bilateral intraventricular hemorrhage with extensive right-sided periventricular venous infarction (*arrows*) with hemorrhagic conversion, midline shift and ventriculomegaly. The overlying subcortical white matter and cortex are spared.

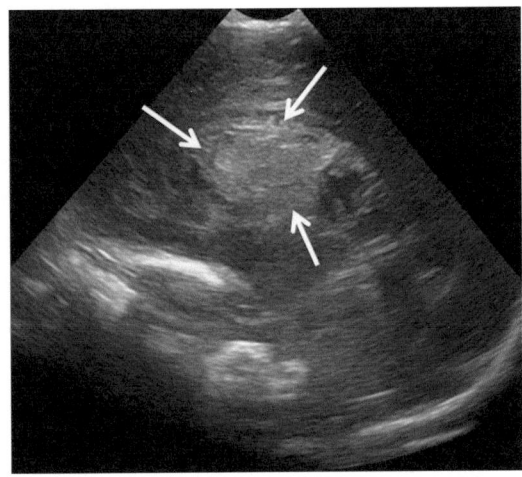

FIG. 7.4. Sagittal image obtained through the anterior fontanelle of a 2-day-old preterm neonate born at 32 weeks of gestation reveals extensive periventricular venous infarction (*arrows*).

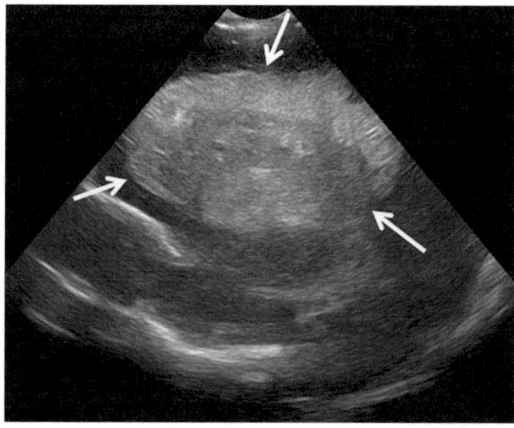

Fig. 7.5. Parasagittal image obtained through the anterior fontanelle of a 2-day-old preterm neonate born at 32 weeks of gestation reveals extensive periventricular venous infarction (*arrows*).

Unilateral Periventricular Venous Infarction (Fig. 7.6)

A 600-g preterm infant was born via C-section for severe pre-eclampsia. On day two of life, he developed worsening acidosis and increased apneic events. A cranial ultrasound performed at that time showed a grade III germinal matrix hemorrhage with right-sided periventricular venous infarction. The following day, reduced left-sided spontaneous movements and severe desaturations were noted and a follow-up head ultrasound was performed.

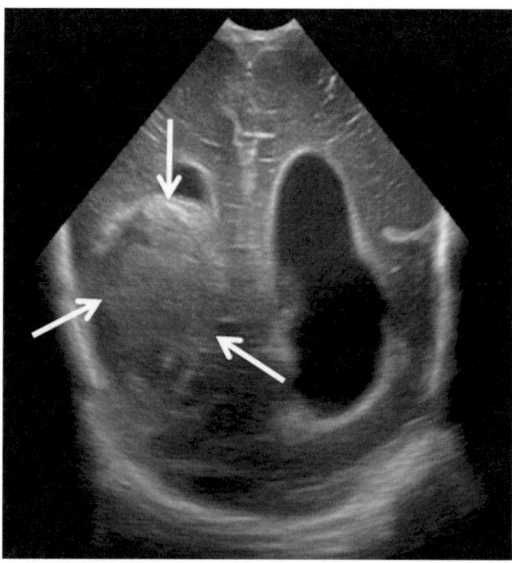

Fɪɢ. 7.6. Coronal image obtained through the anterior fontanelle of a 6-day-old preterm neonate born at 26 weeks of gestation shows a large right parieto-occipital parenchymal hemorrhage (*arrows*) and ventriculomegaly due to mass effect.

References

Abels L, Lequin M, Govaert P. Sonographic templates of newborn perforator stroke. Pediatr Radiol. 2006;36:663–9.

de Vries LS, Roelants-van Rijn AM, Rademaker KJ, Van Haastert IC, Beek FJ, Groenendaal F. Unilateral parenchymal haemorrhagic infarction in the preterm infant. Eur J Paediatr Neurol. 2001;5:139–49.

Dudink J, Lequin M, Weisglas-Kuperus N, Conneman N, van Goudoever JB, Govaert P. Venous subtypes of preterm periventricular haemorrhagic infarction. Arch Dis Child Fetal Neonatal Ed. 2008;93(3):F201–6.

Govaert P. Sonographic stroke templates. Semin Fetal Neonatal Med. 2009;14:284–98.

Huisman TA. Intracranial hemorrhage: ultrasound, CT and MRI findings. Eur Radiol. 2005;15:434–40.

van der Aa NE, Benders MJ, Groenendaal F, de Vries LS. Neonatal stroke: a review of the current evidence on epidemiology, pathogenesis, diagnostics and therapeutic options. Acta Paediatr. 2014;103:356–64.

Chapter 8
Apnea

Neonatal apnea is defined as a pause in breathing that is longer than 15–20 s and is usually associated with bradycardia, cyanosis, or both. Generally, there are two main pathomechanisms for neonatal apnea: central apnea and obstructive apnea. Central apnea is defined as a pause in alveolar ventilation due to a lack of diaphragmatic activity (lack of signal to breathe being transmitted from the brain to the respiratory muscles). On the other side, obstructive apnea is defined as a pause in alveolar ventilation due to obstruction of airflow within the upper airway, particularly at the level of the pharynx. Of course, a combination of both types of apnea may occur.

Multiple etiologies are known for both types of neonatal apnea and include not only neurological causes, but also disorders involving other organs such as the cardiovascular system (e.g., congestive heart failure), pulmonary system (e.g., surfactant deficiency and meconium aspiration), and prenatal exposure to various drugs with transplacental transfer. Here we focus on neurological causes for neonatal apnea. The most common one is apnea related to prematurity and brain stem immaturity (Paul et al. 2009; Theobald et al. 2000). Apneic spells of 10–15 s are present at some time in almost all preterm neonates and are usually associated with a reduction in heart rate. The sudden onset of apneic spells associated with decrease consciousness, particularly in preterm neonates,

© Springer International Publishing Switzerland 2016
A. Poretti, T.A.G.M. Huisman (eds.), *Neonatal Head and Spine Ultrasonography*, DOI 10.1007/978-3-319-14568-6_8

suggests an intraventricular (Owens 2005; Veyrac et al. 2006) or parenchymal hemorrhage (Limperopoulos et al. 2005; Steggerda et al. 2009). Joubert syndrome, a posterior fossa malformation, is a rare cause of neonatal breathing abnormalities in neonates (Poretti et al. 2011).

Apneic spells are an uncommon manifestation of seizures, particularly in preterm neonates, unless they are associated with tonic deviation of the eyes, hypertonia of the body, and clonic/myoclonic limb movements. However, in term neonates apnea may be the only clinical manifestation particularly in epileptic seizures with temporal lobe onset (Cross 2013; Tramonte and Goodkin 2004). In addition, a seizure has to be ruled out in prolonged apneas, particularly if associated with tachycardia.

Differential Diagnosis of Brain Abnormalities Associated with Apnea That May Be Detected by Neonatal Head Ultrasonography

- Prematurity (see Chap. 3)
- Cerebellar hemorrhage
- Intraventricular hemorrhage
- Joubert syndrome (see Chap. 6)

Cerebellar Hemorrhage (Figs. 8.1 and 8.2)

A 5-day-old 28-week gestational age neonate has a sudden increase in number of apneic. On examination, he is noted to have global hypotonia and his anterior fontanelle is tense.

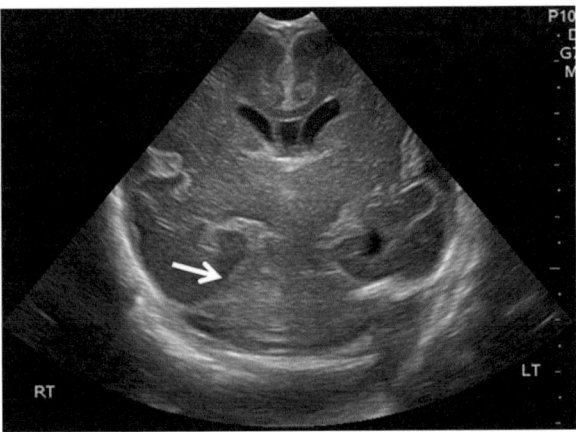

Fig. 8.1. Coronal image obtained through the anterior fontanelle of a 26-week preterm neonate with history of coagulopathy and blood loss requiring multiple fluids shows mildly prominent supratentorial ventricular system, premature cortical and gyral anatomy, and a focal hyperechogenic lesion within the right cerebellar hemisphere concerning for cerebellar hemorrhage (*arrow*).

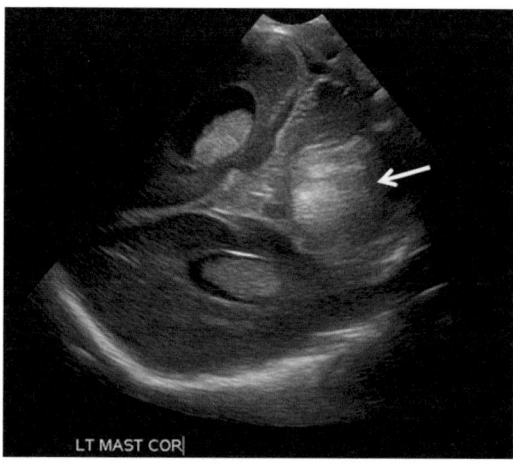

Fig. 8.2. Lateral mastoid approach on coronal view of a 26-week preterm neonate with history of coagulopathy and blood loss requiring multiple fluids clearly shows with higher details the focal hyperechogenic lesion within the right cerebellar hemisphere (*arrow*) that expand into the adjacent cerebellar vermis and is concerning for a cerebellar hemorrhage. This case exemplifies the importance of additional approaches along with the routine anterior fontanelle approach to evaluate the neonatal brain. Especially, mastoid fontanelle and posterior fontanelle approaches are essential to evaluate the posterior fossa structures.

Intraventricular Hemorrhage (Figs. 8.3 and 8.4)

A 3-day-old 26-week gestational age infant has a sudden increase in number of apneic and bradycardic events. On examination, she is noted to have decreased tone from baseline, a lack of eye movements and some fresh blood emerging from her endotracheal tube. Laboratory results reveal a significant decrease in hemoglobin, a profound metabolic acidosis and persistent hyperglycemia.

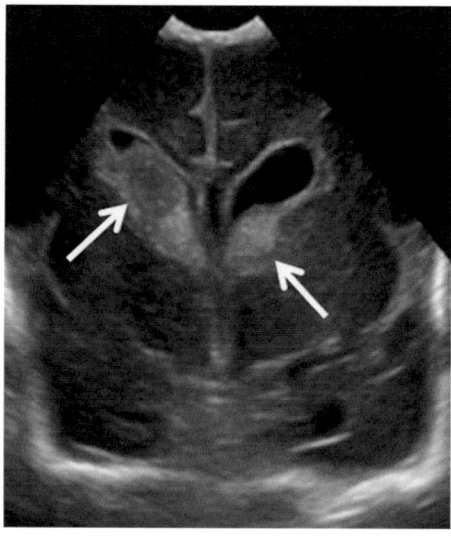

Fig. 8.3. Coronal image obtained through the anterior fontanelle of a 5-day-old preterm neonate born at 26 weeks of gestation with history of acute onset apnea shows a bilateral (*right>left*) grade 3 germinal matrix hemorrhage (*arrows*). Grade 3 germinal matrix hemorrhages are easily identified on head ultrasound by the direct visualization of blood clots within the germinal matrix and the enlarged ventricular system. In addition, ependymal lining is hyperechogenic due to the intraventricular blood products.

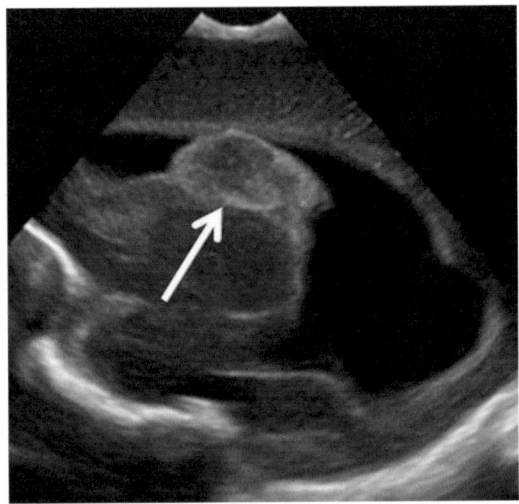

FIG. 8.4. Sagittal image obtained through the anterior fontanelle of a 5-day-old preterm neonate born at 26 weeks of gestation with a history of acute onset apnea shows a focal hyperechogenic hemorrhage in the caudothalamic groove (*arrow*) with moderate ventriculomegaly and hyperechogenic ependymal lining representing a grade 3 germinal matrix hemorrhage.

References

Cross JH. Differential diagnosis of epileptic seizures in infancy including the neonatal period. Semin Fetal Neonatal Med. 2013;18:192–5.

Limperopoulos C, Benson CB, Bassan H, Disalvo DN, Kinnamon DD, Moore M, Ringer SA, Volpe JJ, du Plessis AJ. Cerebellar hemorrhage in the preterm infant: ultrasonographic findings and risk factors. Pediatrics. 2005;116:717–24.

Owens R. Intraventricular hemorrhage in the premature neonate. Neonatal Netw. 2005;24:55–571.

Paul K, Melichar J, Miletín J, Dittrichová J. Differential diagnosis of apneas in preterm infants. Eur J Pediatr. 2009;168:195–201.

Poretti A, Huisman TA, Scheer I, Boltshauser E. Joubert syndrome and related disorders: spectrum of neuroimaging findings in 75 patients. AJNR Am J Neuroradiol. 2011;32:1459–63.

Steggerda SJ, Leijser LM, Wiggers-de Bruïne FT, van der Grond J, Walther FJ, van Wezel-Meijler G. Cerebellar injury in preterm infants: incidence and findings on US and MR images. Radiology. 2009;252:190–9.

Theobald K, Botwinski C, Albanna S, McWilliam P. Apnea of prematurity: diagnosis, implications for care, and pharmacologic management. Neonatal Netw. 2000;19:17–24.

Tramonte JJ, Goodkin HP. Temporal lobe hemorrhage in the full-term neonate presenting as apneic seizures. J Perinatol. 2004;24:726–9.

Veyrac C, Couture A, Saguintaah M, Baud C. Brain ultrasonography in the premature infant. Pediatr Radiol. 2006;36:626–35.

Chapter 9
Microcephaly

Microcephaly is defined as an occipito-frontal circumference of two standard deviations or more below the mean for age, gender, and gestation measured over the greatest frontal circumference. Microcephaly is a rather common finding and may occur in isolation or be associated with other abnormalities. Microcephaly at birth denotes a fundamental impairment in normal prenatal brain development. Neonatal microcephaly may be caused by a myriad of conditions including both genetic and environmental (disruptive) etiologies (Alcantara and O'Driscoll 2014; Ashwal et al. 2009; von der Hagen et al. 2014). Ultrasound is very helpful in detecting the underlying cause of microcephaly as well as following changes/growth of the head size over time.

Genetic causes of neonatal microcephaly include brain malformations such as holoprosencephaly, primary microcephaly, lissencephaly, or schizencephaly (Deeg and Gassner 2010; Deeg 2011; Rios et al. 2012), neurometabolic diseases such as Smith-Lemli-Opitz disease, and chromosomal abnormalities such as trisomy 13 or 18. Environmental causes of neonatal microcephaly include prenatal infections such as cytomegalovirus and rubella (Capretti et al. 2014), drugs with teratogenic/toxic effect such as alcohol, hydantoin, and radiation, and maternal conditions such as poorly controlled diabetes mellitus type 1 or phenylketonuria.

© Springer International Publishing Switzerland 2016
A. Poretti, T.A.G.M. Huisman (eds.), *Neonatal Head and Spine Ultrasonography*, DOI 10.1007/978-3-319-14568-6_9

Differential Diagnosis of Brain Abnormalities Associated with Microcephaly That May Be Detected by Neonatal Head Ultrasonography

–   Holoprosencephaly (see Chap. 11)
–   Lissencephaly
–   Schizencephaly
–   Primary microcephaly
–   Congenital rubella infection
–   Congenital cytomegalovirus infection (see Chap. 4)

Lissencephaly (Figs. 9.1, 9.2, and 9.3)

A full-term infant with a history of polyhydramnios in utero was noted to have mild hypotonia after birth. He was transferred to the intensive care unit for hypoglycemia in the setting of poor feeding and intermittent apneas.

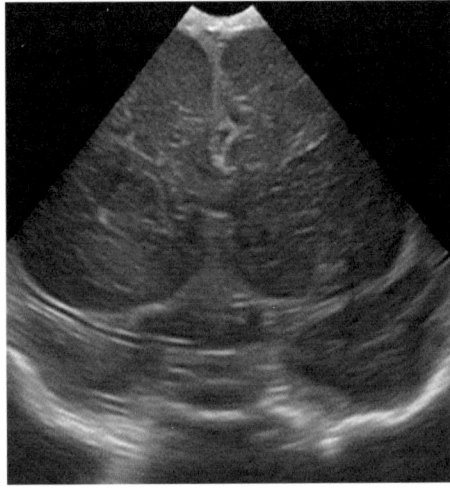

Fig. 9.1. Coronal image obtained through the anterior fontanelle of a 1-month-old infant with lissencephaly shows a smooth brain surface with absent corticomedullary differentiation. A smooth brain is physiologically seen in very preterm newborns, but is abnormal at term.

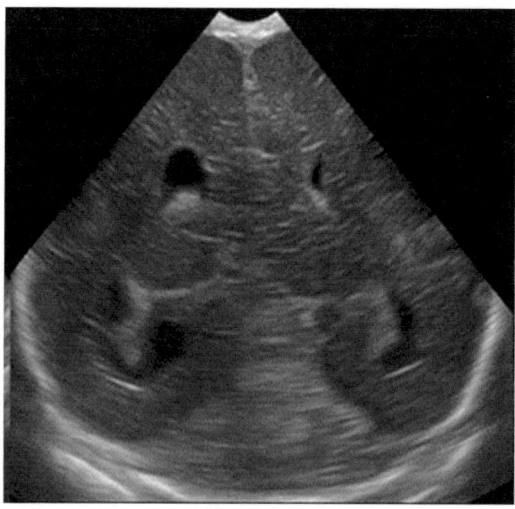

FIG. 9.2. Coronal image obtained through the anterior fontanelle of a 1-month-old infant with lissencephaly reveals a smooth brain surface with absent corticomedullary differentiation. A mild ventriculomegaly is also seen.

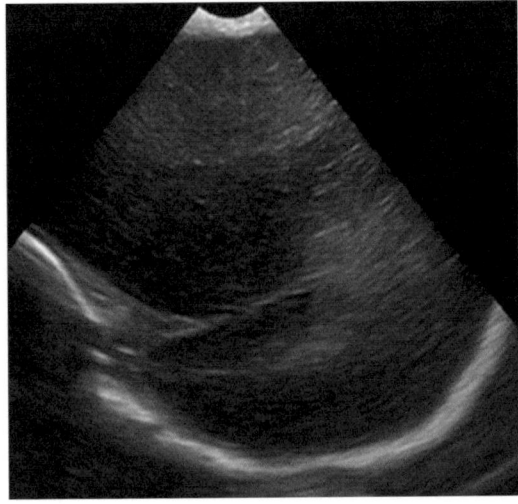

FIG. 9.3. Sagittal image obtained through the anterior fontanelle of a 1-month-old infant with lissencephaly shows a smooth brain surface with absent corticomedullary differentiation.

Schizencephaly (Figs. 9.4 and 9.5)

A full-term infant was noted to have microcephaly at birth and a normal neurologic exam. On the third day of life, the infant had an episode of global atony that was associated with desaturations and tachycardia. Electroencephalography revealed normal background activity with right parietal focal sharp waves.

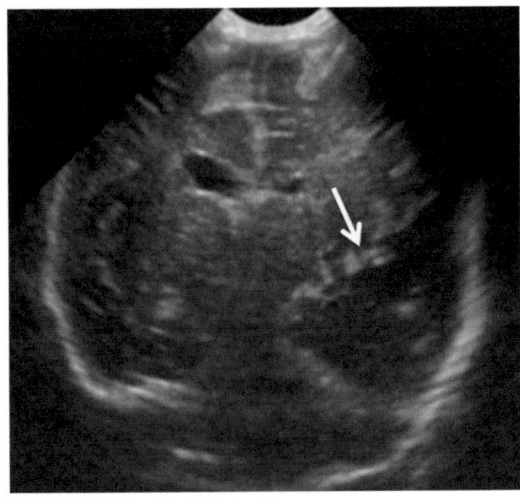

FIG. 9.4. Coronal image obtained through the anterior fontanelle of a 26-day-old term neonate with left-sided temporal schizencephaly shows a left temporal cleft which extends toward the adjacent left lateral ventricle and is lined by thickened, dysplastic cortex (*arrow*).

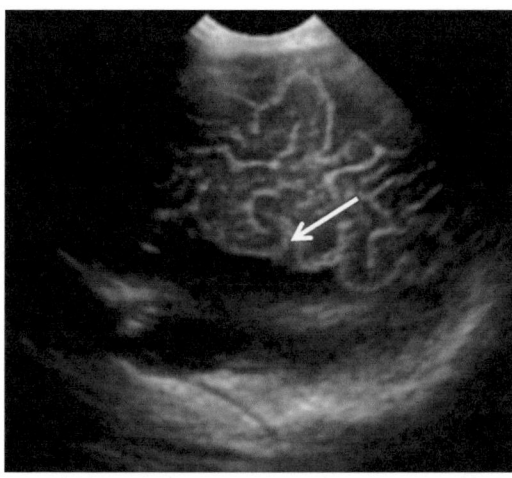

FIG. 9.5. Left parasagittal image obtained through the anterior fontanelle of a 26-day-old term neonate with left-sided temporal schizencephaly reveals a left temporal cleft (*arrow*) extending toward the adjacent left lateral ventricle.

Congential Rubella Infection
(Figs. 9.6, 9.7, and 9.8)

A full-term infant was born to a mother with poor prenatal care. Immediately following delivery, the provider noted lethargy, global hypotonia, irritability, and a full anterior fontanel. Upon crying, the infant arched his back and had extensor posturing of the lower extremities. The infant would also have episodes of profuse sweating and excessive sucking.

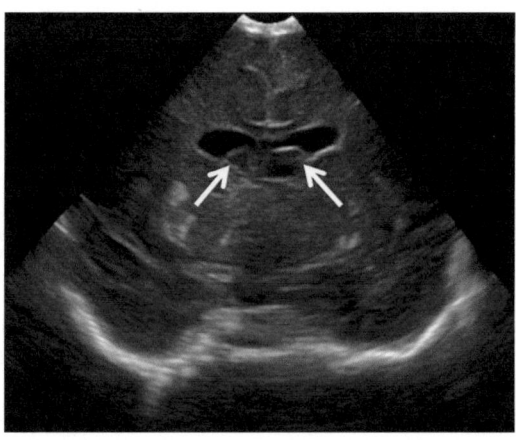

FIG. 9.6. Coronal image obtained through the anterior fontanelle of a 4-day-old term neonate with a history of intrauterine growth restriction, congenital rubella infection, patent ductus arteriosus, and thrombocytopenia shows well-circumscribed intraventricular cysts (*arrows*) bilaterally.

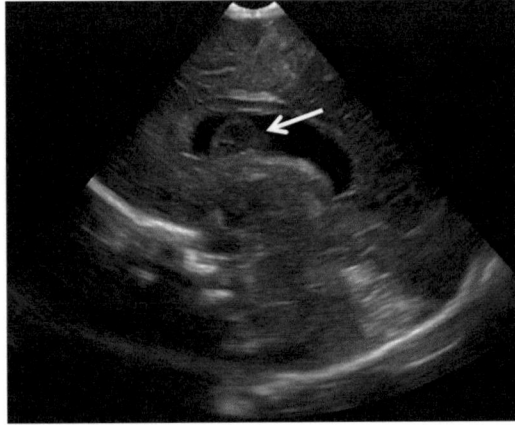

Fig. 9.7. Left parasagittal image obtained through the anterior fontanelle of a 4-day-old term neonate with a history of intrauterine growth restriction, congenital rubella infection, patent ductus arteriosus, and thrombocytopenia reveals a well-circumscribed intraventricular cyst (*arrows*) within the lateral ventricle.

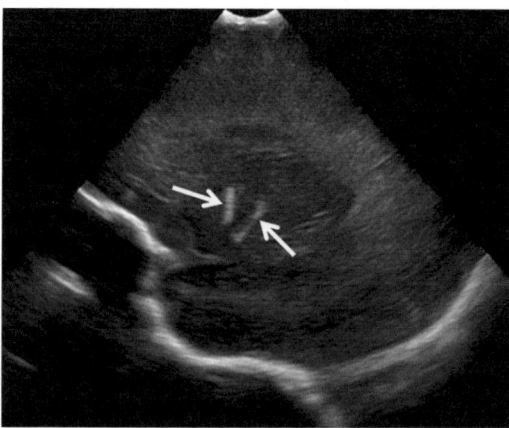

FIG. 9.8. Right parasagittal image obtained through the anterior fontanelle of a 4-day-old term neonate with a history of intrauterine growth restriction, congenital rubella infection, patent ductus arteriosus, and thrombocytopenia shows discrete curve-linear mineralizing vasculopathy (*arrows*) within the basal ganglia that may be seen in congenital infections by rubella, cytomegalovirus, and toxoplasmosis.

References

Alcantara D, O'Driscoll M. Congenital microcephaly. Am J Med Genet C Semin Med Genet. 2014;166C:124–39.

Ashwal S, Michelson D, Plawner L, Dobyns WB, Quality Standards Subcommittee of the American Academy of Neurology and the Practice Committee of the Child Neurology Society. Practice parameter: evaluation of the child with microcephaly (an evidence-based review): report of the Quality Standards Subcommittee of the American Academy of Neurology and the Practice Committee of the Child Neurology Society. Neurology. 2009;73:887–97.

Capretti MG, Lanari M, Tani G, Ancora G, Sciutti R, Marsico C, Lazzarotto T, Gabrielli L, Guerra B, Corvaglia L, Faldella G. Role of cerebral ultrasound and magnetic resonance imaging in new-borns with congenital cytomegalovirus infection. Brain Dev. 2014;36:203–11.

Deeg KH. Sonographic diagnosis of cerebral malformations. Part 3: agenesis of the corpus callosum — migration disorders. Ultraschall Med. 2011;32:128–44.

Deeg KH, Gassner I. Sonographic diagnosis of brain malformations, part 2: holoprosencephaly — hydranencephaly — agenesis of septum pellucidum — schizencephaly — septo-optical dysplasia. Ultraschall Med. 2010;31:548–60.

Rios LT, Araujo Junior E, et al. Prenatal and postnatal schizencephaly findings by 2D and 3D ultrasound: pictorial essay. J Clin Imaging Sci. 2012;2:30.

von der Hagen M, Pivarcsi M, Liebe J, von Bernuth H, Didonato N, Hennermann JB, Bührer C, Wieczorek D, Kaindl AM. Diagnostic approach to microcephaly in childhood: a two-center study and review of the literature. Dev Med Child Neurol. 2014;56:732–41.

Chapter 10
Macrocephaly

Macrocephaly is defined as an occipito-frontal circumference
of two standard deviations or more above the mean for age,
gender, and gestation, measured over the greatest frontal
circumference. Neonatal macrocephaly may be caused by a
myriad of conditions including hydrocephalus (McAllister
2012; Taylor 2001), cerebral edema, and a truly enlargement
of the brain or megalencephaly (Mirzaa and Poduri 2014).

Hydrocephalus describes dilatation of the brain ventricles
and is the most common cause of neonatal macrocephaly.
Occipital and frontal horns are affected first. Changes in the
velocity of cerebral arterial flow may be seen in obstructive
hydrocephalus (Brouwer et al. 2010). Symptoms and clinical
findings of newborns with hydrocephalus include poor feeding, vomiting, irritability, apneic spells, episodes of bradycardia, a bulging anterior fontanelle, and distended scalp veins.
Etiologies of neonatal hydrocephalus include post-
hemorrhagic hydrocephalus, congenital or neonatal infections, malformations of the cerebral/cerebellar morphogenesis
and ventricular system, and, rarely, congenital brain tumors.
Ultrasound is very helpful in detecting hydrocephalus and its
underlying cause as well as following changes in ventricular
size over time.

© Springer International Publishing Switzerland 2016   119
A. Poretti, T.A.G.M. Huisman (eds.), *Neonatal Head and
Spine Ultrasonography*, DOI 10.1007/978-3-319-14568-6_10

Post-hemorrhagic hydrocephalus occur in about 25–35 % of neonates with intraventricular hemorrhage and the incidence is inversely related to the gestational age (Govaert and de Vries 2010). Serial head ultrasonography measurements of the lateral ventricles may play a key role in the early recognition and therapeutic evaluation of post-hemorrhagic hydrocephalus and can be of prognostic value in neonates. In addition, hydrocephalus is a common feature of some brain malformations such as Chiari 2 malformation and Dandy–Walker malformation that may be detected by ultrasonography (Brennan and Taylor 2010). Finally, neonatal hydrocephalus may be also caused by a vascular malformation (e.g., vein of Galen malformation) (Huisman et al. 2010) or an abnormality along the cerebrospinal fluid pathway (e.g., stenosis of the Sylvian aqueduct, that is characterized by a dilatation of the lateral and third ventricles, but normal size of the fourth ventricle).

Differential Diagnosis of Brain Abnormalities Associated with Macrocephaly That May Be Detected by Neonatal Head Ultrasonography

– Post-hemorrhagic hydrocephalus
– Chiari 2 malformation
– Dandy–Walker malformation
– Vein of Galen malformation
– Stenosis of the Sylvian aqueduct

Post-hemorrhagic Hydrocephalus (Figs. 10.1, 10.2, and 10.3)

An infant born at 26 weeks gestational age with a history of grade III intraventricular hemorrhage at day of life three developed a progressively bulging anterior fontanelle over the subsequent 2 weeks. On the most recent exam, the provider noted an upward gaze palsy and widening of the cranial sutures. A graph of the infant's head circumference showed rapid growth that crossed percentile lines.

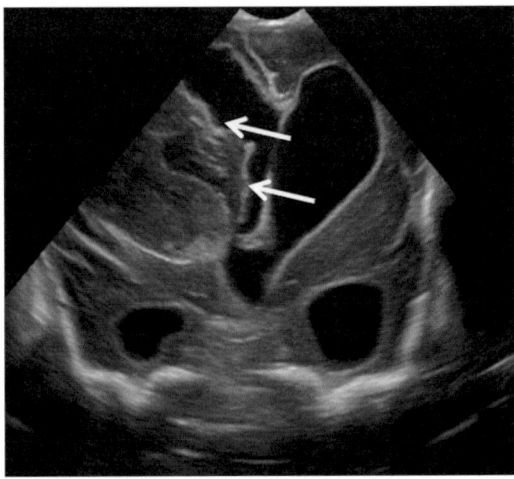

Fig. 10.1. Coronal image obtained through the anterior fontanelle of an 18-day-old preterm neonate born at 25 weeks 5 days of gestational age with a history of intraventricular hemorrhage shows the interval evolution of the intraventricular hemorrhage (*arrows*) associated with severe ventriculomegaly and right-to-left midline shift.

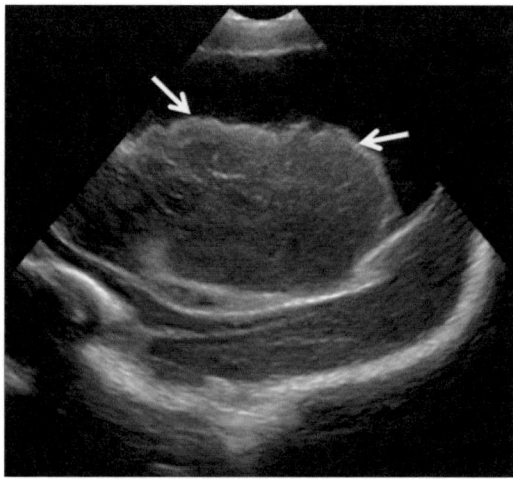

FIG. 10.2. Right parasagittal image obtained through the anterior fontanelle of an 18-day-old preterm neonate born at 25 weeks 5 days of gestational age with a history of intraventricular hemorrhage shows the interval evolution of the intraventricular hemorrhage (*arrows*) associated with severe ventriculomegaly.

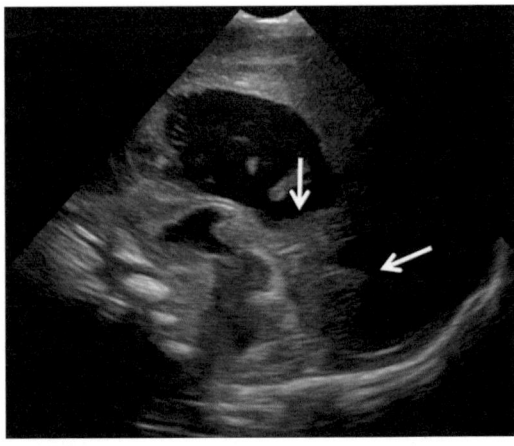

FIG. 10.3. Sagittal image obtained through the anterior fontanelle of an 18-day-old preterm neonate born at 25 weeks 5 days of gestational age with a history of intraventricular hemorrhage shows the interval evolution of the intraventricular hemorrhage (*arrows*) associated with severe ventriculomegaly.

Chiari 2 Malformation (Figs. 10.4, 10.5, and 10.6)

A full-term infant was born to a mother with poor prenatal care via precipitous delivery. During the resuscitation, the provider found a sac of tissue protruding from the infant's midline lower back, hypotonia of the lower limbs, and macrocephaly. Subsequently the infant was noted to have stridor, periods of apnea, and poor feeding.

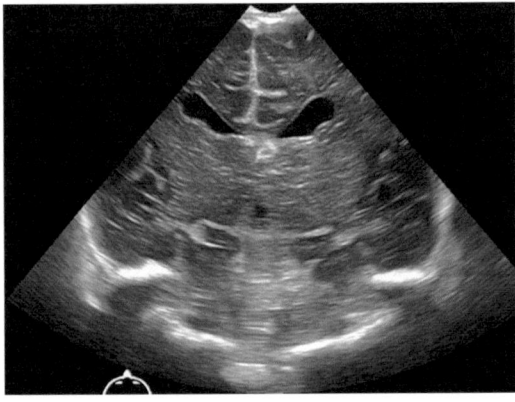

FIG. 10.4. Coronal image obtained through the anterior fontanelle of a term neonate with non-skin covered myelomeningocele and Chiari 2 malformation reveals a small posterior fossa and a moderate ventriculomegaly.

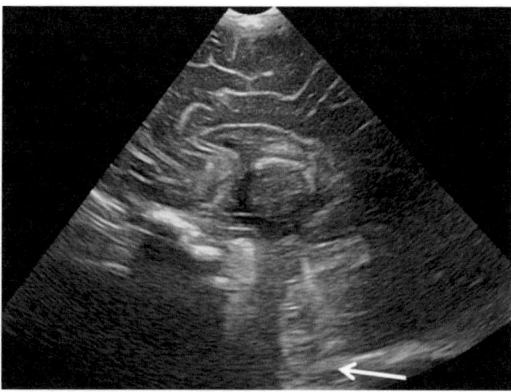

F<small>IG</small>. 10.5. Sagittal image obtained through the anterior fontanelle of a term neonate with non-skin covered myelomeningocele and Chiari 2 malformation shows a small posterior fossa, low insertion of tentorium cerebelli, and partial herniation of the cerebellar vermis into the cervical spinal canal (*arrow*).

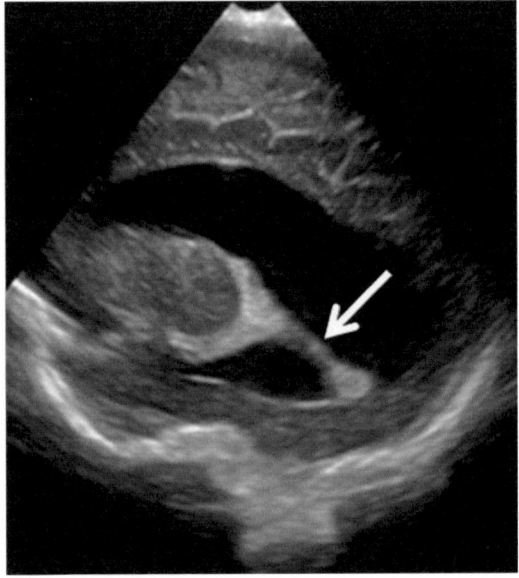

FIG. 10.6. Parasagittal image obtained through the anterior fontanelle of a term neonate with non-skin covered myelomeningocele and Chiari 2 malformation reveals a dangling choroid plexus (*arrow*) within the occipital horns of the lateral ventricles.

Dandy–Walker Malformation (Figs. 10.7, 10.8, and 10.9)

A full-term infant was born to a mother who received prenatal care at a different hospital. After delivery, she reported that the prenatal ultrasound showed "fluid on the brain" but does not know any more information. The infant was noted to be macrocephalic with an otherwise normal neurologic examination. Cardiac examination is significant for a harsh, blowing holosystolic murmur.

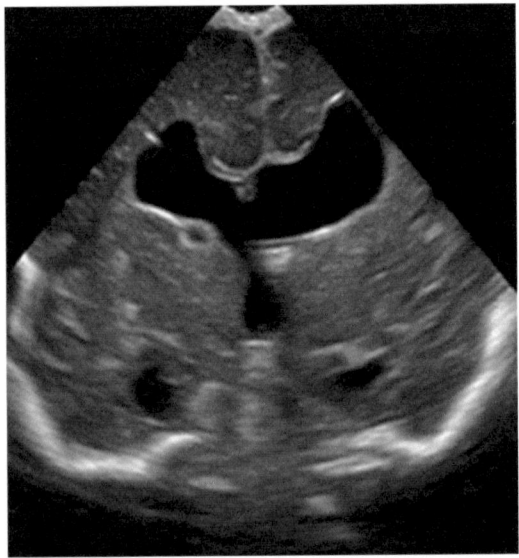

FIG. 10.7. Coronal image obtained through the anterior fontanelle of a 1-month-old baby with Dandy–Walker malformation shows parallel configuration of lateral ventricles due to a thin and malformed corpus callosum and a marked hydrocephalus.

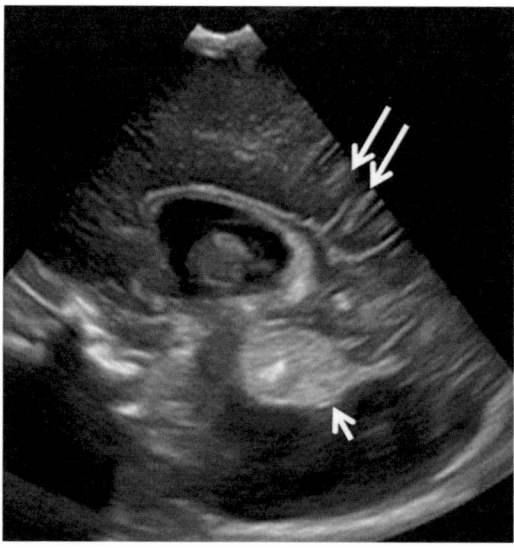

Fig. 10.8. Sagittal image obtained through the anterior fontanelle of a 1-month-old baby with Dandy–Walker malformation shows a hyperechogenic upward rotated, hypoplastic cerebellar vermis (*short arrow*), a cystic enlargement of the fourth ventricle, a thin and malformed corpus callosum and the mesial sulci are radiating from the region of the third ventricle (*long arrows*).

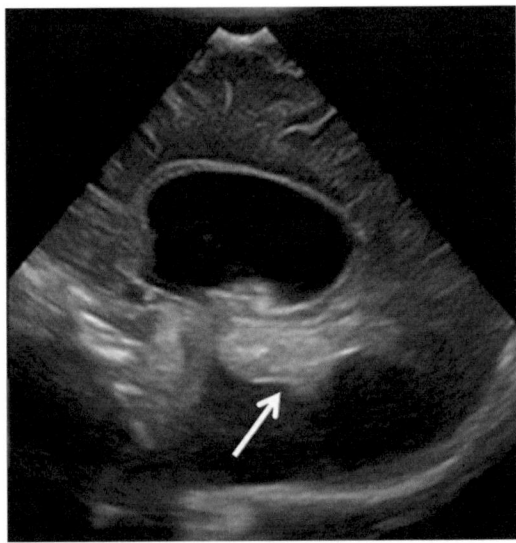

Fig. 10.9. Sagittal image obtained through the anterior fontanelle of a 1-month-old baby with Dandy–Walker malformation shows a hyperechogenic upward rotated, hypoplastic cerebellar vermis (*arrow*), a cystic enlargement of the fourth ventricle and significant hydrocephalus.

Vein of Galen Malformation (Figs. 10.10, 10.11, and 10.12)

A 36-week-old infant was born via induced vaginal delivery for concern for hydrops fetalis and right heart failure on prenatal echocardiography. The infant required immediate intubation due to poor respiratory effort. Macrocephaly and a dilated scalp vein were noted on exam. Post-natal echocardiogram showed suprasystemic pulmonary hypertension with right-to-left shunting as well as aortic dilatation.

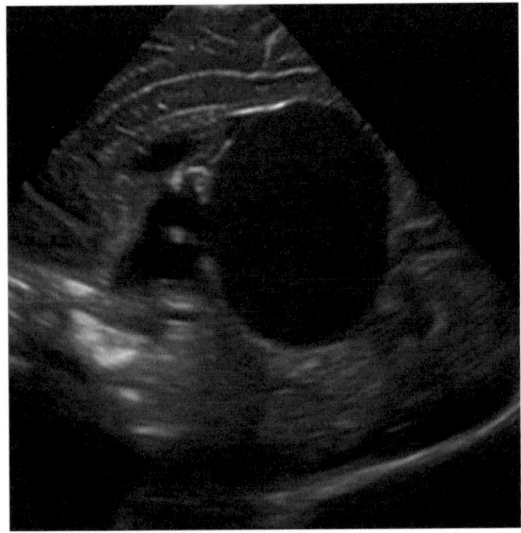

Fig. 10.10. Sagittal image obtained through the anterior fontanelle of a 3-day-old term neonate with prenatally diagnosed vein of Galen malformation shows a large hypoechogenic well-circumscribed dilatation of the vein of Galen that compresses the dorsal mesencephalon.

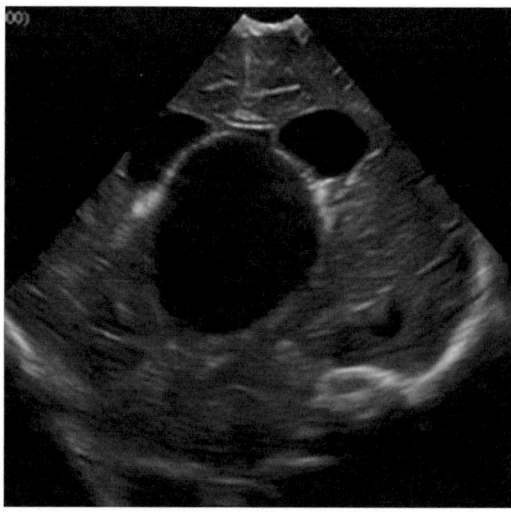

FIG. 10.11. Sagittal image obtained through the anterior fontanelle of a 3-day-old term neonate with prenatally diagnosed vein of Galen malformation shows a large hypoechogenic well-circumscribed dilatation of the vein of Galen which compresses the dorsal mesencephalon and results in a moderate supratentorial ventriculomegaly.

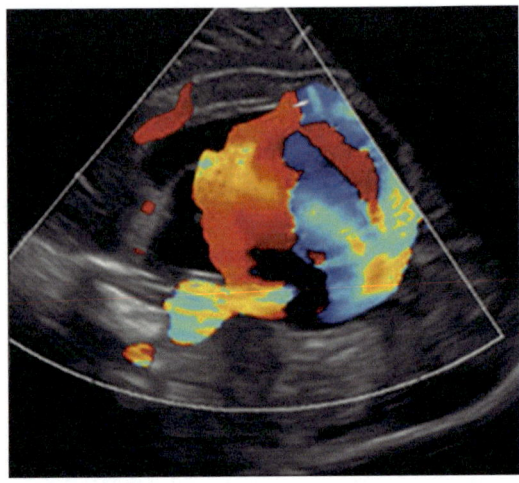

FIG. 10.12. Sagittal color-coded image obtained through the anterior fontanelle of a 3-day-old term neonate with prenatally diagnosed vein of Galen malformation reveals a turbulent flow within the dilated vein of Galen.

References

Brennan CM, Taylor GA. Sonographic imaging of the posterior fossa utilizing the foramen magnum. Pediatr Radiol. 2010;40: 1411–6.

Brouwer MJ, de Vries LS, Pistorius L, Rademaker KJ, Groenendaal F, Benders MJ. Ultrasound measurements of the lateral ventricles in neonates: why, how and when? A systematic review. Acta Paediatr. 2010;99:1298–306.

Govaert P, de Vries LS. An atlas of neonatal brain sonography. London: Mac Keith; 2010. p. 46–9.

Huisman TA, Singhi S, Pinto PS. Non-invasive imaging of intracranial pediatric vascular lesions. Childs Nerv Syst. 2010;26:1275–95.

McAllister JP. Pathophysiology of congenital and neonatal hydrocephalus. Semin Fetal Neonatal Med. 2012;17:285–94.

Mirzaa GM, Poduri A. Megalencephaly and hemimegalencephaly: breakthroughs in molecular etiology. Am J Med Genet C Semin Med Genet. 2014;166C:156–72.

Taylor GA. Sonographic assessment of posthemorrhagic ventricular dilatation. Radiol Clin North Am. 2001;39:541–51.

Chapter 11
Craniofacial Dysmorphic Features

A dysmorphic feature is defined as a body characteristic that is abnormally formed. Dysmorphic feature may occur as isolated findings in otherwise normal individuals or in combination as part of genetic syndromes (Allanson et al. 2009a; Hennekam et al. 2013). A high number of craniofacial dysmorphic features have been described (Allanson et al. 2009b). Some of the craniofacial dysmorphic features are associated with brain malformations such as holoprosencephaly (Deeg and Gassner 2010; Hahn and Barnes 2010), lissencephaly (Guerrini and Dobyns 2014), and agenesis or dysgenesis of the corpus callosum (Atlas et al. 1985; Palmer and Mowat 2014). These brain malformations may be detected by head ultrasonography.

Differential Diagnosis of Brain Malformation Associated with Craniofacial Dysmorphic Features That May Be Detected by Neonatal Head Ultrasonography

- Holoprosencephaly
- Agenesis or dysgenesis of the corpus callosum
- Lissencephaly (see Chap. 4)
- Joubert syndrome (see Chap. 6)
- Dandy-Walker malformation (see Chap. 10)

© Springer International Publishing Switzerland 2016   139
A. Poretti, T.A.G.M. Huisman (eds.), *Neonatal Head and Spine Ultrasonography*, DOI 10.1007/978-3-319-14568-6_11

Holoprosencephaly (Figs. 11.1, 11.2, 11.3, and 11.4)

A full-term infant was delivered to a diabetic mother with no prenatal care. Exam was significant for hypotelorism, a flattened nasal bridge, median cleft lip and palate and a single median maxillary incisor. Laboratory studies revealed serum sodium of 160 mEq/L and very low thyroid-stimulating hormone (TSH).

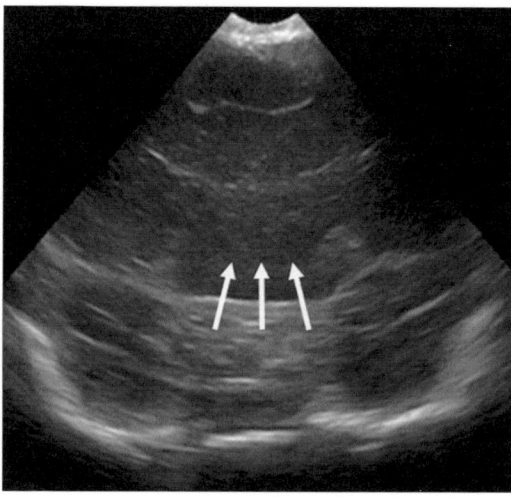

FIG. 11.1. Coronal image through the anterior fontanelle of a 14-day-old term neonate with semilobar holoprosencephay shows fusion of the frontal lobes (*arrows*).

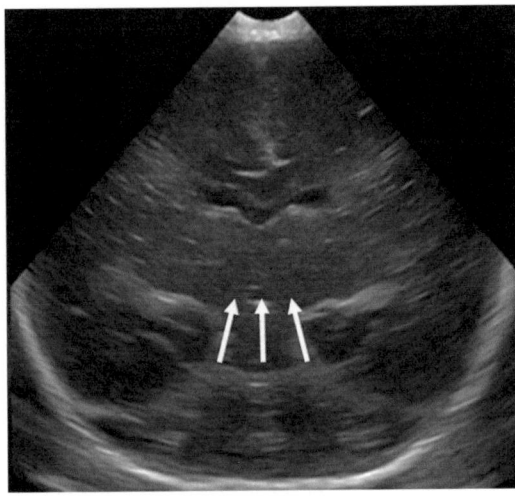

F<small>IG</small>. 11.2. Coronal image through the anterior fontanelle of a 14-day-old term neonate with semilobar holoprosencephay shows fusion of the frontal lobes (*arrows*) and absence of the anterior corpus callosum.

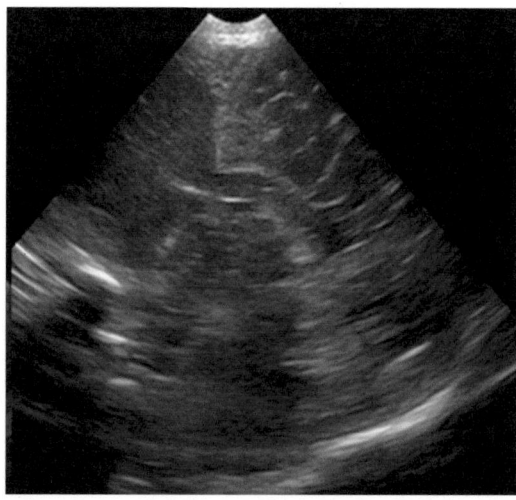

FIG. 11.3. Sagittal image through the anterior fontanelle of a 14-day-old term neonate with semilobar holoprosencephay shows absence of the anterior corpus callosum. In addition, the posterior part of the telencephalon is splitted with a normal appearing posterior corpus callosum.

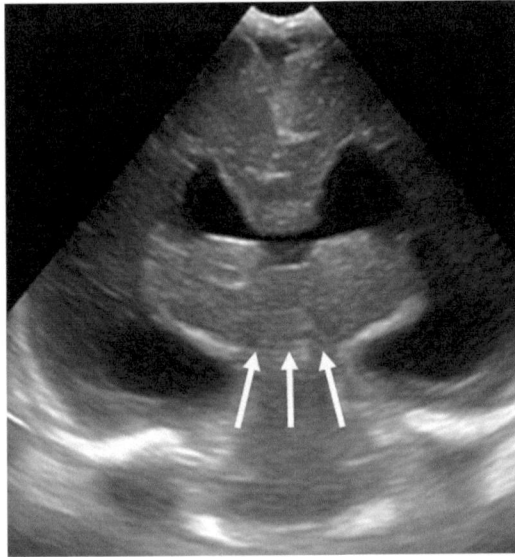

FIG. 11.4. Coronal image through the anterior fontanelle of an 18-day-old term neonate with semilobar holoprosencephaly shows partially fusion of the thalami (*arrows*), absence of the anterior corpus callosum, and moderate ventriculomegaly.

Agenesis of the Corpus Callosum
(Figs. 11.5 and 11.6)

A full-term infant was born to a mother who had limited prenatal care and urine toxicology positive for benzodiazepines. On exam, the infant was noted to have a small philtrum, thin vermilion, and small palpebral fissures. He was also found to be microcephalic and small for gestational age.

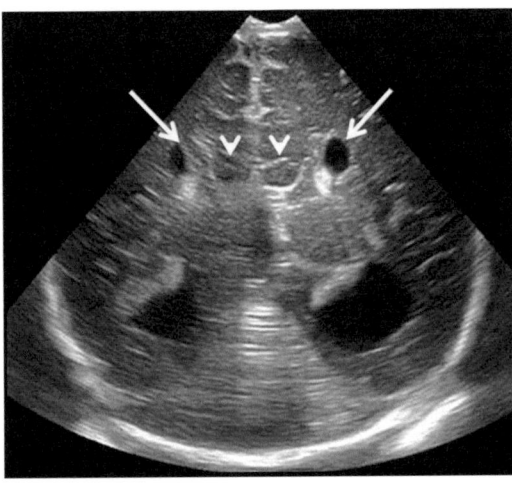

FIG. 11.5. Coronal image through the anterior fontanel of 1-day-old term neonate with prenatally diagnosed ventriculomegaly and craniofacial dysmorphic features shows the characteristic "Texas Longhorn" configuration of the lateral ventricles (*arrows*), which are mildly lateralized and enlarged. In addition, malrotation of the bilateral cingulate gyrus is noted (*arrowheads*).

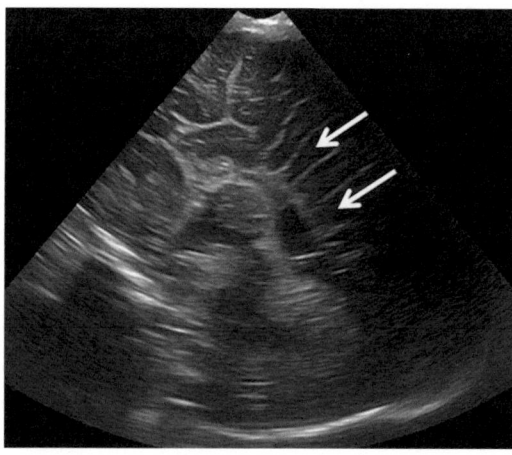

Fig. 11.6. Sagittal image through the anterior fontanel of 1-day-old term neonate with prenatally diagnosed ventriculomegaly and craniofacial dysmorphic features reveals absence of the corpus callosum and radiation of the mesial sulci (*arrows*) from the region of the third ventricle.

References

Allanson JE, Biesecker LG, Carey JC, Hennekam RCM. Elements of morphology: introduction. Am J Med Genet A. 2009a;149A:2–5.

Allanson JE, Cunniff C, Hoyme HE, McGaughram J, Muenke M, Neri G. Elements of morphology: standard terminology for the head and face. Am J Med Genet A. 2009b;149A:6–28.

Atlas SW, Shkolnik A, Naidich TP. Sonographic recognition of agenesis of the corpus callosum. AJR Am J Roentgenol. 1985;145:167–73.

Deeg KH, Gassner I. Sonographic diagnosis of brain malformations, part 2: holoprosencephaly—hydranencephaly—agenesis of septum pellucidum—schizencephaly—septo-optical dysplasia. Ultraschall Med. 2010;31:548–60.

Guerrini R, Dobyns WB. Malformations of cortical development: clinical features and genetic causes. Lancet Neurol. 2014;13:710–26.

Hahn JS, Barnes PD. Neuroimaging advances in holoprosencephaly: refining the spectrum of the midline malformation. Am J Med Genet C. 2010;154C:120–32.

Hennekam RCM, Biesecker LG, Allanson JE, Hall JG, Opitz JM, Temple IK, Carey JC, Elements of Morphology Consortium. Elements of morphology: general terms for congenital anomalies. Am J Med Genet A. 2013;161A:2726–33.

Palmer EE, Mowat D. Agenesis of the corpus callosum: a clinical approach to diagnosis. Am J Med Genet C. 2014;166C:184–97.

Chapter 12
How to Perform a Neonatal Spine Ultrasonography Study and Normal Spine Ultrasound in the Neonate

For an informative, diagnostic ultrasonography (US) study of the neonatal spine, an up-to-date, technologically advanced, US unit is essential (Figs. 12.1 and 12.2). A high-frequency 7–12 Mhz linear transducer is usually used and provides high-quality longitudinal and transverse images of the entire spine from the craniocervical junction to the coccyx (Ladino Torres and DiPietro 2014). Ultrasound images are typically acquired with the neonate in lateral decubitus or prone position. A slight flexion of the spine allows a better window over the midline between the posterior spinous processes.

The normal spinal cord is hypoechoic with a hyperechoic dorsal and ventral surfaces as well as a central complex that results from the interface of the myelinated ventral white commissure and the central end of the anterior median fissure (Nelson et al. 1989). The cerebrospinal fluid (CSF) around the spinal cord is anechoic, while the nerves in the subarachnoid space are hyperechoic. The size and shape of the spinal cord is variable depending of the level: larger and oval at the cervical, lower thoracic, and thoracolumbar level, while smaller and round at the upper and middle thoracic and lower lumbar level, where it gradually forms the conus medullaris (Unsinn et al. 2000). In neonates, the position of the tip of the conus medullaris is normally located between L1 and L2 and may occasionally extend to the superior aspect of L3 (Fig. 12.3) (DiPietro 1993; Unsinn et al. 2000).

© Springer International Publishing Switzerland 2016   149
A. Poretti, T.A.G.M. Huisman (eds.), *Neonatal Head and Spine Ultrasonography*, DOI 10.1007/978-3-319-14568-6_12

Distally, the filum terminale extends from the tip of the conus medullaris to the caudal end of the sacral spinal canal. The filum terminale has a homogenous mildly hyperechoic signal and a normal thickness of 1–2 mm (Dick et al. 2002).

When performing neonatal spine ultrasonography, it is important to be aware of normal variants such as the ventriculus terminalis and filar cyst. The ventriculus terminalis is a persistent fetal terminal ventricle in the conus medullaris due to incomplete regression of the caudal spinal cord. On ultrasonography, it appears as focal widening of the central echo complex of the conus medullaris and is essentially similar to hydromyelia, but limited to the conus (Lowe et al. 2007). The filar cyst is a cystic midline structure seen within or adjacent/inferior to the filum terminale located caudally to the conus medullaris. Usually, it has an ovoid form and it is best seen with high-frequency transducers (Irani et al. 2006).

In addition to gray-scale anatomical imaging, images of the spine vasculature may be sampled using Doppler US (Fig. 12.4).

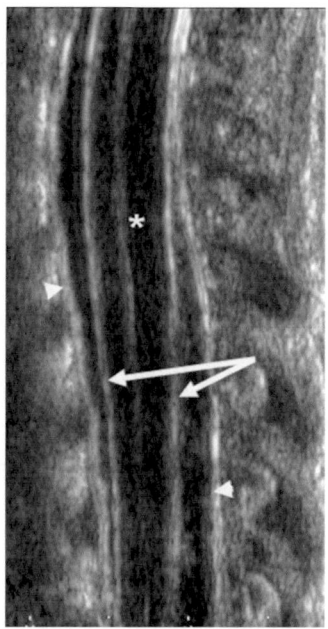

FIG. 12.1. Normal neonatal spine sonography. Sagittal US image of the thoracic spine shows the normal hypoechoic spinal cord with a hyperechoic dorsal and ventral surface (*arrows*) and central complex (*asterisk*). The spinal cord is surrounded by hypoechoic cerebrospinal fluid. Note the hyperechoic dura (*arrowheads*).

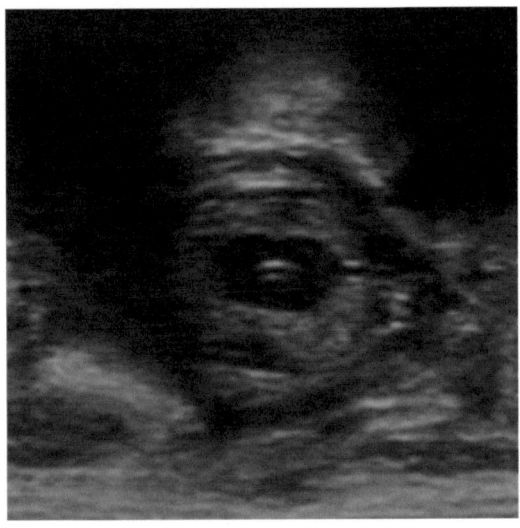

FIG. 12.2. Axial ultrasonography image of a normal lumbar spinal cord.

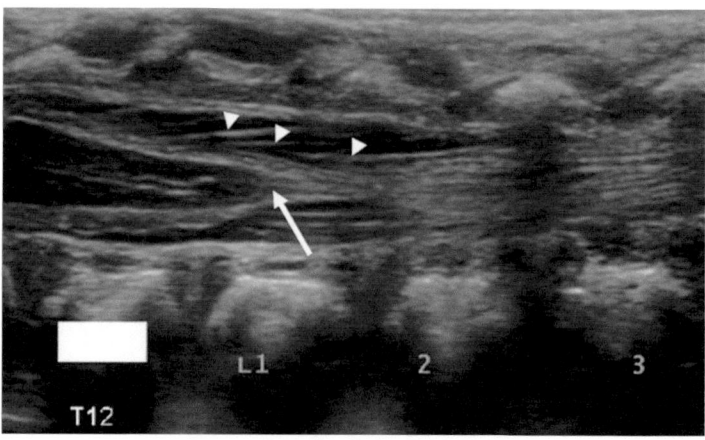

FIG. 12.3. Normal neonatal spine sonography. Sagittal image of the lumbar spine shows the normal hypoechoic spinal cord with hyperechoic dorsal and ventral surface and central complex. The spinal cord is surrounded by hypoechoic cerebrospinal fluid and fine hyperechoic nerves (*arrowheads*) in the subarachnoid space. Note the normal smooth tapering of the conus medullaris (*arrow*), which is normally positioned at the level of L1. Note the hyperechoic dura.

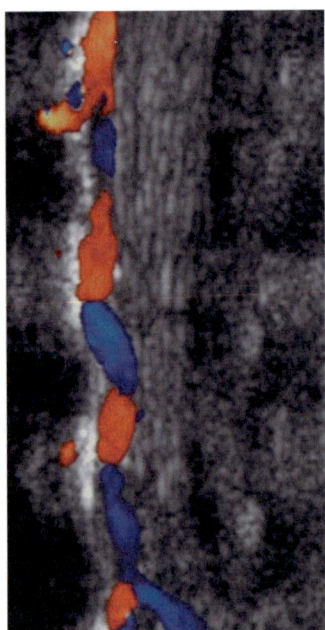

Fig. 12.4. Longitudinal color-coded Doppler sonography of the normal spinal cord allows the evaluation of the spine vasculature. *Red coding* indicates flow towards the US probe, *blue* relates to flow away from the US probe.

References

Dick EA, Patel K, Owens CM, De Bruyn R. Spinal ultrasound in infants. Br J Radiol. 2002;75:384–92.

DiPietro MA. The conus medullaris: normal US findings throughout childhood. Radiology. 1993;188:149–53.

Irani N, Goud AR, Lowe LH. Isolated filar cyst on lumbar spine sonography in infants: a case-control study. Pediatr Radiol. 2006;36:1283–8.

Ladino Torres MF, DiPietro MA. Spine ultrasound imaging in the newborn. Semin Ultrasound CT MR. 2014;35:652–61.

Lowe LH, Johanek AJ, Moore CW. Sonography of the neonatal spine: Part 1. Normal anatomy, imaging pitfalls, and variations that may simulate disorders. Am J Roentgenol. 2007;188:733–8.

Nelson MD, Sedler JA, Gilles FH. Spinal cord central echo complex: histoanatomic correlation. Radiology. 1989;170:479–81.

Unsinn KM, Geley T, Freund MC, Gassner I. US of the spinal cord in newborns: spectrum of normal findings, variants, congenital anomalies, and acquired diseases. Radiographics. 2000;20:923–38.

Chapter 13
Neonatal Spine Abnormalities

Spinal dysraphia is defined as a defect of posterior neuropore closure (Copp et al. 2013). Spinal dysraphia may be skin-covered or non-skin-covered. Non-skin-covered spinal dysraphia is usually diagnosed prenatally and is associated with intracranial abnormalities (Chiari 2 malformation) (Huisman et al. 2012). Skin-covered spinal dysraphia is usually less apparent at birth and commonly brought to attention by the presence of abnormalities in the overlying skin (such as an abnormal tuft of hair, pigmentation, a sinus opening, or a mass). Neonatal spine ultrasonography may clarify the underlying anatomical changes and provide a precise diagnosis (Ladino Torres and DiPietro 2014).

Types of Spinal Dysraphia That May Be Detected by Neonatal Spine Ultrasonography

- Myelomeningocele (non-skin-covered spina bifida)
- Diastematomyelia (skin-covered spina bifida)
- Lipomyelomeningocele (skin-covered spina bifida)
- Dorsal dermal sinus
- Caudal regression syndrome

© Springer International Publishing Switzerland 2016   157
A. Poretti, T.A.G.M. Huisman (eds.), *Neonatal Head and Spine Ultrasonography*, DOI 10.1007/978-3-319-14568-6_13

Myelomeningocele (Figs. 13.1 and 13.2)

A full-term infant was delivered by a C-section after the pre-natal diagnosis of a non-skin-covered lumbar myelomeningocele. Exam showed flaccid legs, absent Achilles reflexes, and bilateral clubfoot.

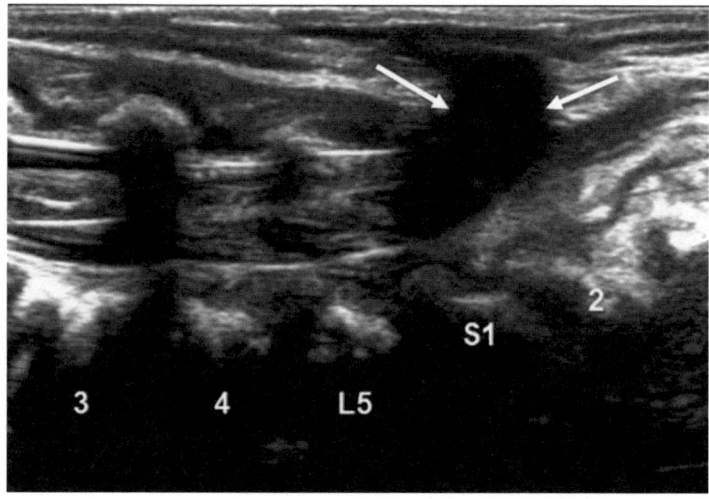

FIG. 13.1. Sagittal image of the lumbar spine shows a non-skin-covered myelomeningocele (*arrows*).

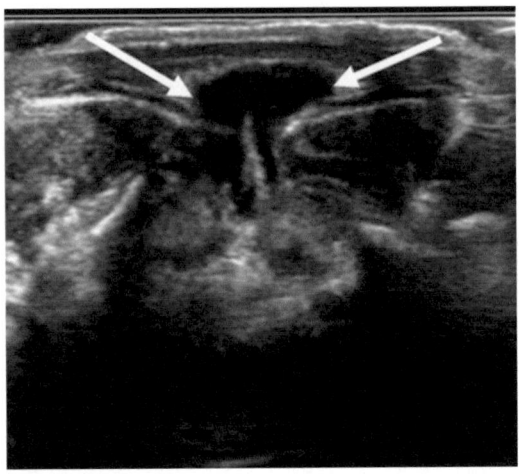

FIG. 13.2. Axial image of the lumbar spine shows a non-skin-covered myelomeningocele (*arrows*).

Diastematomyelia (Fig. 13.3)

A full-term infant showed an abnormal tuft of hair over the lumbar spine in the midline.

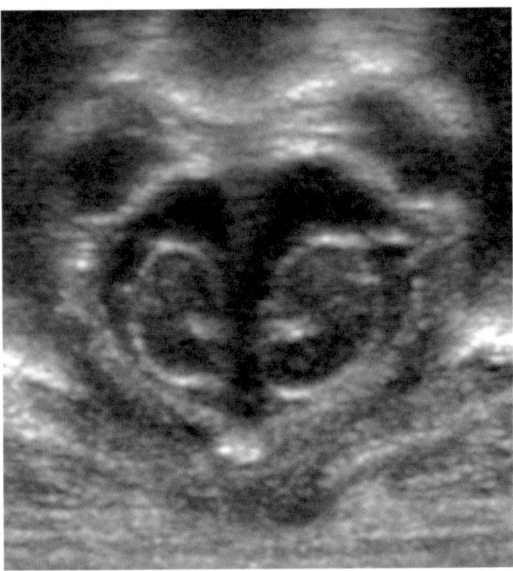

FIG. 13.3. Axial image of the lumbar spine of a neonate with diastematomyelia shows 2 hemicords within the dural sac and an osseous septum in the midline.

Dorsal Dermal Sinus (Fig. 13.4)

A full-term infant showed a port wine stain over the lumbar spine in the midline.

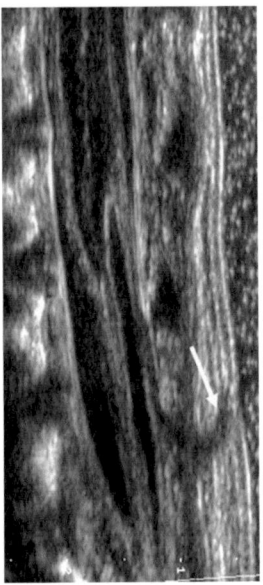

FIG. 13.4. Sagittal image of the lumbar spine of a neonate with dorsal dermal sinus shows the hypoechoic sinus tract (*arrow*) connecting the intraspinal space with the epidermis.

Caudal Regression Syndrome (Fig. 13.5)

A full-term infant presented after birth small, flaccid legs.

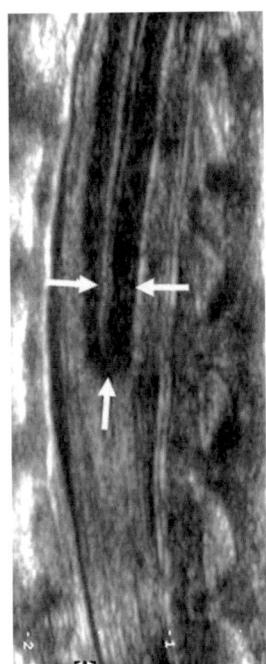

FIG. 13.5. Sagittal image of the lumbar spine of a neonate with caudal regression syndrome shows a blunted appearance of the conus medullaris (*arrows*) with associated short spinal cord with absent caudal portions.

References

Copp AJ, Stanier P, Greene ND. Neural tube defects: recent advances, unsolved questions, and controversies. Lancet Neurol. 2013;12: 799–810.

Huisman TA, Rossi A, Tortori-Donati P. MR imaging of neonatal spinal dysraphia: what to consider? Magn Reson Imaging Clin N Am. 2012;20:45–61.

Ladino Torres MF, DiPietro MA. Spine ultrasound imaging in the newborn. Semin Ultrasound CT MR. 2014;35:652–61.

Index

© Springer International Publishing Switzerland 2016
A. Poretti, T.A.G.M. Huisman (eds.), *Neonatal Head and
Spine Ultrasonography*, DOI 10.1007/978-3-319-14568-6

Made in the USA
Monee, IL
10 May 2026